Ana Paula Cavalcante dos Santos

RA: a study of semen donation in Brazil

Ana Paula Cavalcante dos Santos

RA: a study of semen donation in Brazil

A study on semen donation in the Brazilian context

ScienciaScripts

Imprint

Cover image: www.ingimage.com

This book is a translation from the original published under ISBN 978-3-330-76599-3.

Publisher:
Sciencia Scripts
is a trademark of
Dodo Books Indian Ocean Ltd. and OmniScriptum S.R.L publishing group

120 High Road, East Finchley, London, N2 9ED, United Kingdom
Str. Armeneasca 28/1, office 1, Chisinau MD-2012, Republic of Moldova, Europe
Managing Directors: Ieva Konstantinova, Victoria Ursu
info@omniscriptum.com

Printed at: see last page
ISBN: 978-620-8-53652-7

DEDICATORY

I dedicate this work to my son Bernardo, for everything he represents in my life, for everything he has made me learn, rethink, change, be, not be...

Also, to all those who, in some way, have come into contact with human reproductive technologies.

And to all the generous people.

ACKNOWLEDGEMENTS

To my advisor, Professor Luiz Antonio de Castro Santos, for his wisdom, competence, humour, presence, sincerity, friendship, affection, support and everything else we exchanged during our time together. In my opinion, our meeting was a pure gift!

To my co-supervisor, Professor Maria Helena Rodrigues Navas Zamora, for being a wonderful person, for the knowledge she shared with me and for her support.

CAPES, for the aid granted, without which this work would not have been carried out.

To Vera Feher Brand, for her indispensable help in recruiting subjects.

To the professors who took part in the qualifying exam: Márcia Arán, Fátima Cecchetto and Carlos Henrique Assunção Paiva.

To the thesis defence committee: Fátima Cecchetto, Carlos Henrique Assunção Paiva, Cid Manso and Lina Faria.

To the professors who participated as alternates: Benilton Bezerra, Alba Zaluar, Maria Elizabeth Ribeiro dos Santos and Osnir Claudiano Jr.

To my teacher and supervisor Jane Russo, for everything I received from you.

Professor Maria Andrea Loyola, for her valuable advice on the subject of this study.

To the IMS professors from whom I learnt so much: Sérgio Carrara, Fabíola Rohden, Laura Moutinho, Benilton Bezerra, Ruben de Mattos, Maria Andréa Loyola, Márcia Arán, Madel Luz, Alba Zaluar, Malu Heilborn.

The friends I met at IMS: Angélica Motta and Vanessa Rangel. My lifelong friends: Christianne, Kika, Collins, Grynea, Ivanete, Marilza and those from "IEVE".

To the secretariat staff, who were always kind and helpful: Márcia, Sílvia Regina, Simone, Eliete, Marco, Elir, Ana Silvia, as well as the IT and library staff.

To my mum, Margarida, for taking care of Bernardo with such dedication and affection every time I needed it. For being my friend as well as my mum.

To my siblings Paulo, Pedro and Adriana, for everything we've exchanged.

To the *Sousa Costa family.* Ivanete, Leonardo, Leozinho and Ana Paula, for welcoming my son with such affection and generosity, which facilitated the writing of this thesis.

To Marilena Jamur, for her precious help in the first steps of my academic life: *unforgettable.*

Writing about co-operation and solidarity means writing about rejection and mistrust at the same time. Solidarity involves individuals ready to suffer for the benefit of a wider group and their expectation that each member of that group will do the same for them. It's difficult to talk about these issues from a distance. They touch on intimate feelings of loyalty and sacredness. Anyone who has accepted trust, asked for sacrifices or voluntarily made them knows the power of the social bond.

Mary Douglas

SUMMARY

SANTOS, Ana Paula Cavalcante dos. *Assisted reproduction: a study on semen donation in the Brazilian context.* 2010. 222f. Thesis (Doctorate in Collective Health) - Institute of Social Medicine, Rio de Janeiro State University, Rio de Janeiro, 2010.

This study aims to investigate the factors that motivate men to donate gametes, anonymously and free of charge, to a semen bank, with the aim of procreating infertile people who undergo assisted reproduction treatments. The material researched points to the fact that both the practice and the donors are usually associated with utilitarianism, pecuniary gain and deviant behaviour, and even some of the agents found it difficult to admit to being altruistic. The phenomenon could be explained by various historical and cultural factors. However, based on a set of interviews conducted with donors and the theory of the gift, it was found that, for part of the group, the experience of donation involved conflicts that were overcome in order to fulfil their life goal, or "life mission". In these terms, and according to the results of the research, we can say that semen donation is part of the gift sphere.

Keywords: Assisted reproduction. Semen donation. Gift.

SUMMARY

INTRODUCTION

Human reproductive technologies are medical procedures that work in favour of procreation, both in the sense of contraception (family planning, for example) and conception, with the aim of "solving" male and female infertility problems and fulfilling the ideals of paternity and maternity. This study focuses on conceptive reproductive technologies.

This medical speciality is part of a multifaceted field, intricately delineated and difficult to enter, situated between debates and disputes, in which cultural, ethical, moral, religious, sexual, social and other issues converge. These questions focus on how these technologies are being used, as well as how they are being directed at the public. In this sense, the field has attracted a great deal of interest from various disciplines besides medicine, such as law, psychology, psychoanalysis, anthropology, sociology and biology, among others (MOURA; CENEDEZE, 2001; MELAMED; QUAYLE, 2006; STRATHERN, 2005a, LUNA, 2002, ALLEBRANDT; MACEDO, 2007; PASSOS, 2007).

Inaugurated in the second half of the last century, conceptive technologies have been the subject of debate in various social spheres, due to the fact that they introduce a clear interference in phenomena that have been perceived as "natural", promoting constant re-significations of the nature/culture categories (LUNA, 2002, 2004 and 2007). Thus, old notions about family, kinship, maternity, paternity and conception have been rethought with the introduction of situations such as: pregnancy in the absence of sexual intercourse; the conception of children using gametes donated anonymously; the birth of artificially conceived babies in families made up of homosexuals, where the biological mother is the partner of the gestational mother; *post-mortem* paternity, pregnancy during the menopause, among many other cases. (PASSOS, 2003; PASSOS, 2007; MOURA, 2007; COSTA, 2002, 2004, 2006).

Specifically in Brazil, since its introduction, the practice has remained more focused on the specialisation of professionals abroad; the techniques used are similar to those applied in developed countries; and the frequent technological innovations are quickly transposed as marketable techniques in professional practice, almost always in the private sector (CORRÊA, 2001; ALLEBRANDT, 2008). This means that professionals in the field seem to be more focused on their technical-professional development and less engaged in expanding scientific knowledge regarding the effectiveness of treatments and the impacts they have on physical and psychological health, as well as on the social lives of their users and society itself, something that is reflected both in the ambiguity of the criteria adopted to assess the effectiveness of these technologies, as well as in the irregularities identified in the records of procedures carried out in the period.

Another striking feature of the field is the interest it arouses in the media (CORRÊA, 2001; RAMIRÉZ-GÁLVEZ, 2002). In the early days of the introduction of these technologies in Brazil, in 1990, the soap opera *Barriga de aluguel was* shown on Rede Globo de Televisão, one of the country's most representative broadcasters, which presented the drama experienced by an infertile couple after the birth of their baby, conceived using two ART techniques: *in vitro* fertilisation (IVF) and surrogate motherhood. At the time, the soap opera caused a huge stir, which led to the topic quickly becoming popular throughout the country.

A few decades on, the subject is still a constant subject of interest in fiction and the media. Leaving aside the articles on the subject that have been published in other mass media (newspapers, magazines, *websites,* etc.), last year alone, in 2009, the same broadcaster aired three "heavyweight" programmes.), last year alone, in 2009, the same broadcaster aired three "major" programmes that dealt with the subject: the sitcom *A grande família,* which aired a few episodes about "surrogacy"; the soap opera *Negócio da China,* which had as one of the main pillars of the work the birth of one of the protagonists through heterologous artificial insemination; and the prime-time *soap opera Caminho das Índias*, which again brought to the fore the issue of a successful single woman's pregnancy, which materialised through artificial insemination with donor semen (IASD). Since controversy and sensationalism are the norm, the figure of the donor (who is anonymous in "real life") was introduced into the plot to claim his right to recognition of paternity.

It was interesting to note that the last chapter of this work of fiction dealt with another situation involving the donation of spermatozoa, but with the appeal of popular comedy. From the flat where a family of dubious character lived, belonging to the upper echelons of society, there was the sound of a crowd shouting: "Daddy, daddy, daddy...!". At that moment, when he became aware of the crowd gathered at the entrance to the building and realised what it represented, the father revealed to his wife and son that in his youth he had to resort to semen banks as a way of surviving.

More recently, starting in 2010, the soap opera *Escrito nas estrelas (Written in the Stars)* was broadcast by Rede Globo in the eighteen o'clock slot. The main theme presented by the plot is life after death, from which arises a situation of *post-mortem* insemination related to the main character.

I believe that if, on the one hand, the public learns about infertility treatment techniques through the media, which in turn popularises and even trivialises them, on the other hand, in many cases there seems to be a lack of knowledge about the limitations, complexity, risks, failures and social effects that these techniques produce (RAMIRÉZ-GÁLVEZ, 2002).

The interest aroused by these technologies and the way in which the field is configured, in its various spheres, is not accidental and can be justified by the lack of competent legislation regulating conceptive technologies (CTs), since at the moment, standardisation has been exercised by the actions and interference of the medical sphere, where power over the practices in question is also centred (LEITE, 1995; MOURA; CENEDEZE, 2001; DINIZ, 2003; SILVA; LOPES, 2008). These technologies have been governed by a Resolution of the Federal Council of Medicine (CFM), which provides professionals and clients with some guidelines for the operation of assisted reproduction (ART), but which would not have the autonomy to deal with the countless issues that can result from this process and, on some points, diverges from the legislation in force in the country, regarding the right of every individual to know their biological origins, as well as the recognition of paternity.

The effects of AR procedures can affect the health of the body, and can also touch on central ethical and moral issues, issues which, in a way, shape the ways of living in our societies, giving meaning to what is right or wrong, permitted or forbidden, which can probably produce conflicts in various areas (SALÉM, 1995). In an effort to adapt these reproductions to the social environment, artifices have been created, such as the obligation to be free and anonymous in more controversial procedures (ALLEBRANDT, 2008), and these very artifices can produce new controversies.

Conceptive reproductive technologies (CRTs) have another point of tension, which makes studying the subject an additional challenge: having to circumvent the state of anonymity that surrounds the entire field. Anyone who is involved in any of the sectors of artificial procreation can easily perceive the aura of concealment present in the environment, whether in person or virtually, in contact with those involved in the practice, or even in the style of the material used to publicise infertility treatment services. Similar experiences were reported by researchers Marilena Corrêa (2001), Naara Luna (2007), Débora Allebrandt (2008) and Fernanda Bittencourt Vieira (2008).

Everything to do with assisted reproduction is covered by a kind of masking, invisibility, secrecy and silence. So researching the subject means having to break through this barrier. Furthermore, there is frequent opposition to the intention to legislate and impose limits on these practices, with the argument that the act constitutes an illicit invasion of the subjects' privacy and "right to procreate", as well as an affront to the freedom of research (SALÉM, 1995).

This thesis presents a study on one of the most controversial forms of reproductive technology: that which uses gametes donated by third parties in artificial insemination. Donation rules vary from country to country (LUNA, 2004; ALLEBRANDT, 2008). Gamete extraction methods vary between the sexes, which both reinforces and deconstructs notions we have about the nature/culture dyad (HAIMES, 1993; LUNA, 2002). Thus, the entire process of heterologous assisted reproduction is mediated by a semen bank in the case of male reproductive cells, by the body of professionals in the case of female reproductive cells and, in all cases, by the public and private institutions where the treatment is being carried out (ALLEBRANDT, 2008; COSTA, 2002, 2006).

Recently, more precisely fifteen years ago, the first semen bank was set up in Brazil, in the city of São Paulo. Since then, countless donations have been made and several babies have been born as a result. During this period, not many studies have dealt with the subject of "gamete donation", or have had contact with the donor subject. Since heterologous assisted reproduction is kept absolutely secret and identities anonymous, the individuals seem to be kept in the same absolute secrecy and anonymity. However, such a rule does not provide knowledge of the field, a survey of issues arising from the technique in question, nor does it portray the degree of agreement or disagreement of the subjects involved with the criteria adopted.

In close proximity to this form of reproduction, some questions can be asked: how does the family that opted for heterologous insemination deal with the figure of the donor, the biological father or mother of their child? What kind of interference does the "presence" of the donor generate within these families? Should the fact be exposed or, on the contrary, hidden? How does or will the person generated through donated gametes deal with their life story? What kind of relationship does the donor have with their anonymous biological child? Do all parties agree to the rules of gratuitousness and anonymity required by current regulations?

After coming into contact with the field of TCs and male gamete donation, my study focused on the factors related to the motivation of Brazilian men to donate sperm to a semen bank. The research was based on the theory of the gift, with two main authors as theoretical references: the anthropologist and sociologist Mareei Mauss (1974), who inaugurated and systematised studies on the subject in his *Essay on the Gift,* and the sociologist Jacques Godbout (1999), who continued the work in his work *The Spirit of the Gift.*

The theory of the gift deals with an understanding of the constitution of social life through constant giving and receiving, based on a tension between obligation and spontaneity, whose system is organised in a particular way in each situation and group. This theoretical framework has contributed greatly to this research.

This thesis is divided into five chapters. The first looks at the field of conceptual reproductive technologies. I begin by presenting the field itself, which has been labelled multifaceted, alluding to the intertwining of diverse phenomena. Next, I address the topic of gamete donation in the Brazilian context, and then deal with issues relating to the semen bank: history, function, services provided and the donation process. Finally, I present some of the discussions about ART legislation at national and international level.

The second chapter presents the social implications of assisted reproduction, which both deconstruct and reinforce Western notions of family, kinship, sex, gender and "race", initially going through the themes of social medicalisation and the desire for offspring, which are observed in most societies. Medicalisation and the desire for offspring are phenomena that have been analysed as some of the driving forces behind human reproduction and, consequently, conceptive technologies.

The third chapter presents the theory of the gift, starting with Mauss' analyses. This is followed by some considerations on the author's ideas, based on the thoughts of other intellectuals such as Claude Lévi-Strauss and Pierre Bourdieu. I end with the theory of the modern gift, developed by the aforementioned Jacques Godbout.

In the fourth chapter, conceptive reproductive technologies are placed under the focus of the gift, from which this medical speciality can be analysed from opposing sides. In the academic world of the humanities and social sciences, the idea of linking these technologies to the commercial sector is commonplace, where everything and everyone works in a utilitarian way. However, I propose analysing these techniques from another direction: as a system of gifts, where all the agents act in favour of generating life, the genuine gift, the baby.

The fifth chapter presents the field study and discussions of some pertinent issues relating to the motivation for semen donation, based on the interviewees' testimonies and the national and international literature survey, such as: the importance of generosity; the relevance of descent; the difficulties in experiencing the donation process and the need to overcome them in order to realise its objective; the resistance to attributing altruism, and the Western social constructs of sex and gender; the belonging of semen donation to the sphere of gift.

My interest in the impact of technology on human life has always been present in my career as a researcher. During my master's degree, I dedicated myself to studying the profound and significant changes that individuals and communities have undergone as a result of the recent introduction of technology into modern societies. Computer-mediated psychotherapy was the topic I chose to research.

During my doctorate in Public Health, I came into contact with topics that deal with the association between technology and health, such as conceptive technologies. From then on, my interest in learning about heterologous assisted reproduction developed and my curiosity turned towards making this subject my object of study.

CHAPTER 1

HUMAN REPRODUCTIVE TECHNOLOGIES

Reproductive technologies are a set of procedures in human reproductive medicine that produce conception independently of sexual intercourse. Initially called artificial reproduction, due to its links with technology, genetics and molecular biology, the set of techniques aimed at solving cases of biological or social infertility has *come* to be called *assisted reproduction* (AR), so that the medical speciality that manipulates and "generates" human life is kept as close to the natural as possible, keeping it as far away as possible from the coldness and artificiality to which technology is generally linked (PASSOS, 2007).

In the past, RA was a medical speciality that received little prestige and credibility in the professional world. However, with the passage of time, this practice has become surrounded by high technology, lucrative procedures and numerous interests. Associations between specialists, entrepreneurs and the pharmaceutical and laboratory industries are a fact, from which professionals are provided with the means and materials to make "dreams" come true. Nowadays, the importance that these techniques occupy is the result of the convergence between the credibility of scientific knowledge and the appeal directed at the feasibility of realising the desire for a biological child (CORRÊA 2001; ALLEBRANDT, 2008).The field encompasses countless issues ranging from cloning to surplus embryos, from the desire for offspring to surrogate motherhood, from heterologous artificial insemination to social paternity, from homosexual individuals' access to assisted reproduction to the re-signification of notions of family and kinship, from the reproductive medicine trade to the insertion of the speciality into gift systems, among many others. This chapter will present some reflections on some of the main themes that permeate conceptive reproductive technologies: gamete donation; the medicalisation of human reproduction; the desire for offspring; the characteristics of the practice in Brazil; the semen bank; the laws that regulate CRTs; their ethical and social implications; the changes produced in conceptions of family, kinship, maternity and paternity, as well as the reinforcement of other notions such as "race", sex and gender.

1.1 Outlining a multifaceted field

The emergence of human reproductive technologies is the result of closer ties between the medical field and technological progress, with both conception and contraception being developed at the same time. Contraceptive reproductive technologies work in favour of family planning, i.e. postponing or avoiding pregnancy. Conceptive technologies aim to treat situations of human infertility, male and/or female, with the aim of realising the desire for children on the part of couples or individuals who are unable to reproduce naturally, or even when previous treatments with drugs and/or surgical interventions have been unsuccessful. The field is the result of the process of medicalisation of sexuality and reproduction, which has historically constructed notions about the body, sexuality, men, women, pregnancy, childbirth, breastfeeding and childhood, with the function of social normalisation (CORRÊA, 2001; LUNA, 2002; PASSOS, 2007; ALLEBRANDT, 2008).

CRTs are an exercise in the medicalisation of childlessness, which presupposes, according to Marilena Corrêa, "(...) a norm - of motherhood and/or reproduction - whose deviation would be legitimately corrected by means of proposed technological interventions that result in test-tube babies." (CORRÊA, 2001, p. 25). (CORRÊA, 2001, p. 24), which brings us back to the discussion about the "duty" of procreation, observed in various human societies, and whose theme is very fruitful in sociology and anthropology. The evolution of AR has been characterised by constant technological advances associated with legitimised knowledge and techniques. For example, knowledge of anatomical structure has been complemented by advances in endocrinology and pharmacology and, more recently, the practical-theoretical contribution of the field has been expanded by the development of molecular biology (PASSOS, 2007).

Based on Corrêa's definition:

> Assisted reproduction is the term that defines a set of medical and palliative treatment techniques, in conditions of human hypo-infertility, aimed at fertilisation. These techniques, which replace sexual intercourse in biological reproduction, involve the intervention, in the act of fertilisation, of at least a third party, the doctor, and sometimes a fourth, represented by the figure of the donor of human reproductive material. The donation can be of reproductive cells (or gametes), eggs and sperm, or even of embryos that have already been formed; there can also be the temporary donation of a uterus, also known by terms such as uterus loan, uterus rental, surrogate mother and others (CORRÊA, 2001, p. 11-12).

Initially, the practice used very simple procedures based on "timing" sexual intercourse to increase accuracy and the chances of achieving a pregnancy. The technique developed later was artificial insemination, which was overtaken *by in vitro* fertilisation. Since then, technological developments within this branch of medicine have been constant (TAMANINI, 2003; ALLEBRANDT, 2008). Currently, the main therapeutic options that make up the range of reproductive techniques are:

a. **Artificial insemination** (AI) -> a technique in which sperm is deposited at different levels of the female genital tract. It can be carried out in two ways: **intra-cervical artificial insemination** (IC), which is defined as a simple method capable of reproducing the physiological conditions of sexual intercourse. Its indication is restricted to cases where normal intercourse or intra-vaginal ejaculation is impossible (sexual malformation, sexual disorders, ejaculation disorders or impotence), and **intra-uterine artificial insemination** (IU), which is the deposit of capacitated motile spermatozoa (capable of fertilisation, after the semen has been treated in the laboratory) at the bottom of the uterine cavity at the moment of ovulation.

b. *In vitro* **fertilisation** (IVF) -> a technique in which the egg is fertilised by sperm outside the woman's body. For this, the treatment goes through the stages of hormonal hyperstimulation, ovulation monitoring, aspiration of the eggs, their union with previously prepared spermatozoa in specific plates. These are transferred to an oven at 37°C (thirty-seven degrees centigrade) with 5% (five per cent) CO2 (carbon dioxide), which simulates the environment of the fallopian tubes. In this culture medium, the male and female gametes are transformed into embryos, which are transferred to the uterus via a catheter after a few days.

c. **ZIFT** (zygote to fallopian tube transfer) -> is a variation on IVF in terms of the embryo transfer process, which takes place laparoscopically.

d. **GIFT** (gamete transfer to the fallopian tubes) -> is a similar technique to IVF, but the fertilisation process takes place inside the fallopian tubes and not in the greenhouse. Through laparoscopy, the eggs are aspirated and placed in the fallopian tube with the sperm. From there, the fertilisation process takes its natural course.

e. ICSI (intracytoplasmic sperm injection) -> a technique known as micromanipulation, it was first developed in the early 1990s in Belgium with the aim of helping sperm with limited locomotion to fertilise. Using a micro-needle, the healthy sperm is injected directly into the egg, from which the embryo can develop. Its implantation in the fallopian tubes follows the same principles as IVF.

f. **ROSNI** (spermatid nuclear injection) - a technique used when there is a deficiency in the maturation of the spermatozoa, and can be associated with ICSI. The spermatid (the immature form of the spermatozoon, but which contains the genetic load necessary for reproduction) is removed directly from the testicle and used in the same way as the sperm in ICSI, with the aid of a fine needle.

It's worth noting that it's *in vitro* fertilisation (IVF) techniques that allow access both to the development of genetic research with embryos, eggs and sperm, and to new forms of medical practice, such as predictive medicine and its pre-implantation diagnostic methods capable of assessing the risks of transmitting pathologies through genetic tests (TAMANINI, 2003, p. 11-14).

Most of the authors who study human reproductive technologies point to 1978 as the milestone of their introduction onto the world stage, with the birth of the first human baby conceived by in *vitro* fertilisation. Obviously, this successful result was preceded by several other studies (PASSOS, 2007). In Brazil, and throughout Latin America, the birth of the first test-tube baby - Arma Paula Caldeira - took place in 1984, at a time when AR was being widely publicised in the print and electronic media, which promoted the popularisation of the subject throughout the country.

According to Corrêa,

> (...) Popularisation not in terms of the dissemination of scientific knowledge, or access to assisted reproduction techniques, but of the issue itself, which, having definitively invaded the media, has reached the imaginary of human reproduction, with these new technological forms. (CORRÊA, 2001, p. 112).

In line with the author's comments, today, thirty-two years after the spread of CRTs abroad and twenty-six years in Brazil, there are still some gaps within the field and many unanswered questions, or even questions that have not been debated. For example, assisted reproduction is a practice that results in some success, but it is not infallible. In fact, the success rates publicised both by the media and on the *websites of* specialised private clinics are higher than those actually seen, which would portray a kind of "masking" of the reality of the profession (CORRÊA; LOYOLA, 1999).

Furthermore, at the Latin American level, there is a certain lack of interest among professionals in publicising the results obtained through medical practice, or even in standardising them. Brazilian assisted reproduction medical centres are officially linked to the Latin American Registry, which began its activities with data from 1990, on behalf of the International Working Group of Registries in Assisted Reproduction. The clinics joined on a voluntary basis, filling in a standardised form drawn up by the group with a view to a worldwide cooperative approach. It turned out that few Latin American countries took part in the movement and sent in their results (FRANCO JÚNIOR; WEHBA apud CORRÊA, 2001, p. 157-158).

As far as Brazil's participation is concerned, there was partial adherence by AR centres, as well as omissions and flaws in terms of *recording* the application of treatments and the *results* obtained. For example, with regard to egg donation, results are presented for births, but the number of attempts is omitted. Nor is there any information on artificial insemination with donor semen (IASD) - the oldest technique to be disseminated - which, according to figures published in the press, has already produced "two thousand anonymous fathers".[1] (CORRÊA, 2001, p. 158).

Another problem observed in the field is the failure to define the criteria for evaluating assisted reproduction in terms of the universe of patients exposed to the techniques. Brazil follows the pattern of most developed countries, which considers the universe of cases to be the number of positive punctures (fertilisation), which increases the margin of success, and not the number of hyperstimulation cycles started, which would decrease it. In addition, there is another inconsistency when the total number of births is used as a criterion for the results obtained with ART, but the measure of IVF success is based on pregnancy (CORRÊA, 2001).

As for the negative indicators of reproductive technologies, only two aspects are considered in the Brazilian registry: the incidence of ectopic pregnancy and spontaneous abortion, without any other undesirable effects of the practice being analysed or systematised, such as: the risks and complications related to interventions related to IVF, as well as the higher incidence of abortion, ectopic pregnancy, hypertensive and haemorrhagic syndromes resulting from the practice.

Furthermore, the high rates of treatment abandonment are not recorded or evaluated, which seem to occur due to the clash that usually takes place between the expectations about test-tube babies brought up at the first consultation and learning about the practice: the reality of the procedures, the extent of the treatments, their high costs, the need for expensive medicines, the lack of a guarantee of success, among others (ALLEBRANDT, 2008).

Furthermore, the control maintained over frozen embryos, as well as the material stored in semen banks, their use, destination, pregnancy, etc. does not offer total

[1] It should be noted that the figures refer to 1992, which are certainly much higher today.

security to users and donors.

According to the analysis of data collected in interviews conducted by Corrêa,

> (...) there would be a group of specialists, not represented among those interviewed, whose work is not very transparent to their own colleagues, but is very visible in the public media, and another group more concerned with establishing some criteria in the constitution of this new field, which is still full of contradictions of the most diverse kinds (CORRÊA, 2001, p. 163).

Another characteristic of reproductive technologies is the rapid transposition of their techniques from research experiments to marketable treatments, and the central role of the mass media in their dissemination and popularisation. Such treatments tend to be constant targets of media interest, often occupying space in sensationalist news stories, which are dissociated from necessary debates on the subject, whose knowledge and effects are still incipient. This reality contributes to the construction of a collective imaginary that seems to associate AR, which is founded on the pillars of science and technology, with the *status of* "superiority" and legitimacy that both have today (CORRÊA, 2001; RAMÍREZ-GÁLVEZ, 2002).

Débora Allebrandt (2008) carried out a study on assisted reproduction with a focus on the practice of gamete donation, using national and international newspaper reports as a means of collecting data[2] . Although in different ways, it was found that the various reports on the subject of AR revealed the existence of a fascination with these new technologies, which are frightening because of their "artificiality" and enchanting because they make "dreams" come true. According to the author:

> In the midst of reports highlighting ethical conflicts, concerns about the aggressiveness of treatments and warnings about low success rates (especially in England), long stories are told that emphasise the obstacles along the way, but justify the final reward - the longed-for baby (ALLEBRANDT, 2008, p. 41).

According to the researcher, the fascination with the medical speciality is based on two pillars: advances in science and the redefinition of kinship as a consequence of these advances.

As for the introduction of the practice in Brazil, due to changes in the course of public health policies, human reproductive technologies spread nationally in a rather peculiar way compared to other medical specialities. Most of the time, innovation in the

---

[2] The newspapers researched were: *Folha de São Paulo* (Brazil), *Le Monde* (France), *The Guardian* (England) and *The New York Times* (United States).

biomedical field occurred through university and/or public services, due to the high costs of cutting-edge technological research and the concentration of qualified professionals in these places. In contrast, the introduction and development of AR occurred and continues to occur in the private sector, mainly concentrated in private clinics owned and coordinated by specialist doctors (CORRÊA, 2001; TAMANINI, 2003).

The last two decades of the last century saw drastic changes in the course of the history of Brazilian medicine, when the demand for investment in public and university hospitals declined.

> Thus, assisted reproduction did not follow the traditional path: unlike other practices, it arrived in the country almost exclusively through private medicine. In addition to socio-demographic factors and the current state of bankruptcy of public medicine in Brazil, interests linked to private medicine, the production of services and the medical products industry, among others, which were already strongly and difficultly established in the field of reproduction, contributed to this (CORRÊA, 2001, p. 145-146).

According to interviews carried out by the author, it was found that many AR specialists in the private sector maintain links with the public sector in parallel to their private practice, without practising assisted reproduction in public and/or university and research institutions, due to the total lack of physical, material and financial structure, and this was a reality observed in the municipality of Rio de Janeiro. (CORRÊA, 2001, p. 51).

Currently in Brazil, assisted reproduction services are available in the public sector, but in only a few locations and with the same characteristics as decades ago: deficiency in applying all the techniques already established in the private sector; long waiting times between appointments; limiting the number of attempts to get pregnant to pre-established cycles; lack of suitable material for treatments, such as good quality probes for carrying out insemination, for example; the need for users to pay for medicines, generally coming from the less favoured social classes; the impossibility of carrying out tests in good time on site, which requires them to be carried out in private laboratories, among others. (CORRÊA, 2001; ALLEBRANDT; MACEDO, 2007).

Based on the peculiarity of the health services provided by the public sector, the profile of AR users also differs from that of patients in other medical specialities, which seems to transform the first group of subjects into a "differentiated" type of user. The quotes below illustrate this:

> Even in the only partially free service, the professionals don't believe that, in the end, the patients they treat are "really poor". It is true that at the beginning of treatment:
>
> "There's everything. There's everything from the farmer from the countryside who

> comes in flip-flops to the very special couple who have already been treated at other clinics and the staff usually know what's going on" (Doctor).
>
> However, it is possible to say that even though the "free" service seems to cater democratically for everyone, over time, be it because of the waiting list that compromises care for women over 35, or the discovery that it is necessary to get hold of resources and go and get them - in most cases this takes time or effectively becomes an impossibility - it ends up producing a series of sieves in care that lead us to what professionals characterise as a "differentiated" user. (ALLEBRANDT; MACEDO, 2007, p. 22).

With regard to the other characteristics of CRT clients in the public and private sectors, the profile of the majority of patients undergoing fertility treatments is characterised by heterosexual couples belonging to the high income brackets and attending private practices or clinics. As we still don't have definitive legislation on ART in Brazil, the criteria for offering this type of service to clients who don't conform to the ideal of the nuclear family (homosexuals and single women) has always been and still is determined by the medical sphere, based on subjectivity, i.e. moral, ethical and religious values on a personal level. Based on his research, Corrêa reports that, of the total of four,

> [...] Only one doctor in Rio de Janeiro said she was not opposed to the possibility of artificial insemination of single women or women who defined themselves as homosexuals, citing the Resolution of the Federal Council of Medicine, which expressly states in its text that single women should be included among the people who can benefit from these techniques. (CORRÊA, 2001, p. 152).

The researcher analysed this as a legalistic attitude on the part of the doctor, when she relies on a written rule from the CFM, which is of a provisional nature, as well as conveying a certain ambiguity as to the maintenance of her own position on the subject, when she states that "(...) This practice was, however, excluded from her activities at that time, due to the fact that she did not 'feel prepared to respond to this type of demand' and especially due to the absence of psychologists in her clinic 'to help the team deal with these situations'". (CORRÊA, 2001, p. 152).

In another study carried out in Porto Alegre, RS, interviews were conducted with professionals involved in assisted reproduction, totalling thirty-four subjects (doctors, researchers [veterinarians and biologists] and magistrates), in order to find out the group's opinion on access to reproductive technologies for homosexuals and single people. The majority (fifteen respondents) were in favour; eleven respondents were ambivalent, ten of whom focused on the welfare of the child. One interviewee attributed to society the duty to determine what is favourable; three interviewees opposed the issue raised, based on the dictates of the Catholic religion, to which both they and the institution they work for belong. Five interviewees had no opinion (ALLEBRANDT; MACEDO,

2007, p. 16-17).

The experts' stance on single women's access to assisted reproduction services was similar to their stance on homosexual access. Only three subjects were opposed to the group's access to the techniques, and the reason was due to the institutions where they work. One is Catholic-based and therefore opposed to the use of these services by single women. The other does not use donated gametes (ALLEBRANDT; MACEDO, 2007, p.17).

The age group of clients for conceptive technologies, one of the frequent causes of infertility or hypofertility, is over thirty. Based on the sample analysed in a study carried out by Allebrandt and Macedo (2007, p. 21), the age range of users in Porto Alegre would be::. 21), the age range of users in Porto Alegre would be: 34.9% (thirty-four point nine per cent) of women and 24.1% (twenty-four point one per cent) of men are aged between thirty-one and thirty-five; 27.4% (twenty-seven point four per cent) of women and 31.7% (thirty-one point seven per cent) of men are aged between thirty-six and forty and 10.3% (ten point three per cent) of women and 27.6% (twenty-seven point six per cent) of men are over forty-one. The remainder, or 27.4 per cent (twenty-seven point four per cent) of women and 16.5 per cent (sixteen point five per cent) of men are aged between twenty and thirty.

The professional training of Brazilian specialists took place, and still takes place, through exchanges with qualified professionals in assisted reproduction from foreign countries, and with the frequent support of the media, companies and entrepreneurs in the private sector, with the supervision of treatments, the introduction of new techniques and academic events. "[...] These events were organised around foreign doctors who were invited to come to Brazil to introduce a technique and even set up cohorts of patients undergoing IVF techniques to be monitored by Brazilian doctors. [...]" (CORRÊA, 2001, p. 146). On the other hand, foreign doctors, "[...] as well as contributing to the export of these techniques to Brazil, had the chance to expand and reaffirm their prestige in the area and open up another field of experience with this emerging therapy." (Idem). (Idem). Due to the way in which reproductive technologies and professional training have spread in Brazil, the country seems to be almost on a par with developed countries in terms of the availability of certain assisted reproduction medical services.

The dissemination of CRTs and the whole range of possibilities that emerge from the medical speciality have promoted a constant re-signification of the field, as well as producing social impacts that are still little known, which brings us back to the need to promote ethical and bioethical debates in the scientific environment, which should be extended to society. Characterised as multifaceted, difficult to delineate, difficult to insert and crossed by diverse themes, procreation techniques have generated controversies that are present in several countries. Specifically in Brazil, one of the most controversial procedures is heterologous artificial insemination. This is the subject of this study and will be discussed below.

1.2 Gamete donation in the context of Brazilian assisted reproduction

Reproductive cell donation refers to the practice in which a man's or woman's semen or egg is donated, respectively, to infertile individuals (physically or socially) or to couples who wish to become parents, and is used in assisted reproduction procedures. Some considerations should be made about this phenomenon. Firstly, current regulations establish the rules of secrecy through the anonymity of the identities of those involved in this type of procedure and the gratuitousness of the act. Secondly, there are significant differences between egg and semen donations. These dissimilarities both deconstruct and reinforce social notions. They break down ideas about family and kinship, and intensify notions of sex and gender, for example.

The difference between the two types of donation - semen and egg - is that male reproductive cells can be frozen and female reproductive cells, on the other hand, cannot be frozen, which would cause them to rupture. Studies on the subject are ongoing, but freezing techniques have not yet been satisfactorily perfected. For this reason, egg banks have so far been unviable. This factor produces significant differences in donation procedures between the sexes.

The practice of egg donation is relatively recent in the history of assisted reproduction. At the moment, such donations are made "fresh", the procedure is invasive, involves medication and surgery, implies greater physical proximity between donors and recipients at the time of gamete transfer, and poses a risk to the health of those providing the genetic material. It generally takes place as follows: women who have their ovaries stimulated by specific medication to remove eggs for IVF, and who manage to get pregnant, are offered to donate their spare reproductive cells to another woman who needs them and is unable to produce them. In exchange for the eggs provided, the recipient pays for the donor's treatment. In general, the gamete donor is younger and belongs to the less favoured social classes, while the recipient is usually older and more financially well-off. This procedure is known as *shared donation.*

The donor is selected by the medical team so that the identities of the donor and recipient are kept confidential. At this stage of the process, photographs of both parties (donor and recipient) or the recipient couple are used, and the criteria for choosing are:

immunological compatibility between the parties, which is determined by blood tests, and the phenotypic similarity of those involved in the process (COSTA, 2004, p. 3-6).

Semen donation follows a very different path, as sperm collection, on the other hand, does not involve surgical or pharmacological intervention, just sexual intercourse. Nowadays, the freezing of semen has become routine, allowing it to be stored indefinitely, as well as being able to be transported over long distances. For example, in Denmark, a bank specialising in the procedure sends inseminating doses not only to Norwegian clinics, but also to much of the rest of the world (MELHUUS, 2005). In Brazil, the most important semen bank sends the material to practically the entire country.

1.2.1 Semen bank

A semen bank is a place for collecting, storing and distributing properly preserved gametes, with the aim of using them for future pregnancies. The material can be kept for an indefinite period of time, frozen using a technique called *cryotherapy.* During the freezing stage, the sperm is placed in a canister containing liquid nitrogen at minus 196°C and kept at the collection site. It should be emphasised that, due to the resources used in its preservation, the semen can be sent to any location, regardless of distance, as mentioned above.

The services of a semen bank are provided for professionals and institutions specialising in assisted reproduction, as well as for the individual who needs them in the case of fertility preservation. Its users are usually couples whose man has infertility that cannot be treated, or who has a disease that can be transmitted to the baby, such as haemophilia and AIDS, for example. This group also includes single women and homosexuals.

A semen bank carries out activities aimed at:

a. Registration of human reproduction clinics.
b. Recruitment of semen donors.
c. Donor selection and screening.
d. Sperm collection through masturbation, in the epididymis and testicle or through stimulated ejaculation (vibro- or electro-ejaculation).
e. Supply of donor semen to human reproduction services, with seminal processing.
f. Therapeutic semen bank, which stores semen from patients who are going to undergo treatments that pose a risk of infertility, such as: chemotherapy,

radiotherapy, vasectomy, orchiectomy [34], prostate surgery, among others.

g. Storage of patient semen for Fiv treatment.
h. Semen processing aimed at "sperm capacitation" of the spouse's own material (for intrauterine insemination or IVF). This service is generally requested by gynaecology practices or clinics specialising in ART.
i. Spermogram .[5]

There are currently four semen banks in Brazil: two in the city of São Paulo, one in Maringá, Paraná and another in Fortaleza, Ceará[6] . The main one is in São Paulo, in a discreet street in the Jardim Paulista neighbourhood, and is responsible for supplying inseminating material to almost all of the offices, clinics and hospitals specialising in assisted reproduction in the country. In addition to this location, the company also operates in the interior of the state, in the city of Campinas, in partnership with one of the main reproductive medicine clinics: the *Campinas Human Reproduction Centre.*

Its history began at the *Hospital Israelita Albert Einstein*, where its entire structure was set up by a veterinarian, whose training was totally directed towards the field of human artificial insemination, along the lines of the most modern banks specialising in the practice in developed countries. At the beginning of 2008, the hospital decided to limit its services to the medical clinic and stopped providing fertility services. The semen bank continued its previous activities under the same coordination, but in new premises. The other three Brazilian banks are linked to local private human reproduction clinics and are not as representative as the first in providing services related to the supply of male genetic material.

Candidates for donation are recruited through adverts in the media, mainly in a

[3] The epididymis is a small duct that collects and stores the sperm produced by the testicle. It is located behind the testicle, in the scrotum, and flows into the base of the vas deferens, the canal that takes the sperm to the prostate.

[4] Orchiectomy or orchidectomy is the surgical removal of the testicles due to cancer, tumour or other disease affecting the region.

[5] Spermograms are mainly used to assess the seminal glands, fertility and post-vasectomy monitoring, as well as to clear up infections in this area. Physicochemical, microscopic and morphological evaluations of the spermatozoa are carried out, as well as immunological, biochemical and hormonal evaluations.

[6] Details of the aforementioned semen banks: the main one, located in the South Zone of São Paulo, is Pro-Seed, http://www.pro- seed.com.br. The other belongs to the Fertility Clinic, also located in São Paulo - SP, http://www.fertility.com.br. The third semen bank is in Maringá - PR, linked to the Materbaby Clinic, http://www.materbaby.com.br and the fourth Brazilian bank, located in Aldeota, a noble neighbourhood in Fortaleza - CE, belongs to the Conceptus Clinic, at http://www.clinicaconceptus.com.br.

local magazine, and in the bank's *folders*. The publicity material is based on information, the legitimacy of the service, discretion, altruism, the offer of a (non-financial) reward for the act, and a guarantee of ethics, secrecy and privacy for the candidates. It also relies on the donor who is already registered with the company as a promoter of the company's activities in their social cycle.

As for the prerequisites for donating male gametes, the subject must be between the ages of eighteen and forty-one, be in good health, which extends to his ascendants, agree to the rules of anonymity and gratuity, and collect the material. The aim of the prior selection of donors is to avoid the transmission of possible pathologies to offspring, i.e. men with a history of personal or family illnesses are discarded by the semen bank.

In general, the sperm donation process begins with the candidate presenting themselves at the bank's reception desk, where they register using an identification document and providing their personal details. At this stage, the individual receives an identification number that will accompany them until the end of the screening. They are then referred to a doctor for an interview, where they can clarify any doubts and their state of health is investigated. Forms are also filled in to record their main characteristics, such as: height, weight, skin colour, hair colour and texture, eye colour, blood type and Rh factor, marital status, number of children (if any), place of birth, religion, profession, *hobbies*, and the country of origin of their parents and maternal and paternal grandparents. The candidate also answers questionnaires and signs a consent form agreeing to anonymity. The data collected is identified with the numbering provided initially, and recorded in databases.

Once this stage of the donation process is complete, the subject is sent for serological and bacterioscopic tests, from which studies are carried out on diseases such as syphilis, AIDS, hepatitis B and C, among others. Six semen collections are then carried out, scheduled in advance, with intervals of two to five days of sexual abstinence between each one. To collect the sperm, the donor is taken to a private location where various erotic resources are made available, as well as a bottle for storing the material. Afterwards, the samples are frozen separately and kept on *standby* for six months - a quarantine period - until the process is completed. Once the period is up, the donor returns to the semen bank and repeats all the tests initially carried out. If approved, the reproductive cells are made available to potential recipients. On the other hand, if the test results are positive for any pathology, at any time during the donation process, the samples are automatically discarded and the candidate is disqualified as a semen donor.

At the time of fertilisation, the choice of donor is usually made by both the medical team and the recipient(s), or by one party or the other, based on the immunological and phenotypical compatibility of the parties involved. Immunological compatibility is determined by blood tests, and phenotypic compatibility refers to similarities in physical characteristics, which is validated by data provided by the bank on the donor, contained in tables where the subjects are listed by number. The tables are organised in terms of "race", and there are three main ones: Caucasians (whites), Asians (Orientals) and blacks (mulattos and negroes).

The request for the material is made by form to the semen bank, or by the clinic or professional specialising in assisted reproduction. The applicant, whether an individual or a company, must be registered with the company. The bank sends the recipient a bank slip for payment. Once receipt has been confirmed, the canister containing the inseminating dose is sent to the applicant's address by post. It should be noted that this is a procedure adopted by Brazil, which may not be the case in other countries. In the case of the USA, for example, there are *websites* that transact the sperm dose directly with the client (who can be from anywhere in the world), thus excluding the participation of assisted reproduction professionals in the transaction.

According to current regulations on HTs, the act of donation must comply with the criterion of gratuity, i.e. the donor does not receive any kind of payment for the donated material. However, the supply of an inseminating dose nowadays costs the recipient between R$1,000.00 (one thousand reais) and R$1,500.00 (one thousand five hundred reais), according to information provided by the director of the Brazilian semen bank, in an interview with me[7] . The justifications for charging this amount refer to the costs involved in the processes of: collecting the material; culture and storage (which involve state-of-the-art technology); and shipping the sperm. I think that the very maintenance of the semen bank is part of the argument.

The monetary aspect of gamete donation has generated some controversy in academic circles. For several researchers, this factor would de-characterise the speciality and semen donation itself from the category of free practice, as required by current Brazilian legislation. This is exacerbated by the high prices of the treatments and, above all, the fact that the possibility of pregnancy is very small. The next section will deal with the regulation of reproductive technologies. This will be followed by a discussion on the link between ART and the market.

---

[7] The data presented was collected in an interview with the director of the Brazilian semen bank, located in São Paulo - SP, in October 2008. The material is digitally recorded.

1.3 **Legislation**

The way in which assisted reproduction is being regulated varies greatly between countries, which could be explained by historical, cultural and social peculiarities. England, for example, is considered to be the "cradle" of the speciality. As one of the forerunners of CT scans, it made history by "producing" the world's first test tube baby. Throughout its history, the country has stood out for the attention it has always paid to ethical, moral and legal issues related to ART. Accordingly, at the request of the British government, an Interdisciplinary Committee was organised in 1990, coordinated by philosopher Mary Warnock, whose main objective was to establish ethical limits in reproductive practices. The numerous debates, which resulted in the Warnock Report, served as the basis for the drafting of the British legislation that went on to regulate the speciality, dating from the same year, *The Human Fertilisation and Embryology Act* and the creation of the *HFEA - The Human Fertilisation and Embryology Authority* (YVON et al, 2004).

In that country, despite having a specific law and permanent control and surveillance, reproductive technologies have never ceased to generate controversy. As a result of the constant debates on the subject and the valorisation of children's rights, the rule of anonymity in gamete donation was vetoed in 2005, producing changes to the previous legislation. This change was motivated by the right of every person to know their biological origins. According to Jasanoff (2005), England's stance on reproductive practices was one of instability and uncertainty, based on the fact that legislating would be a solution found by the country to minimise the conflicts in which it finds itself immersed.

The US has not enacted a specific law regulating reproductive medicine, due to its strong federal tradition. Legislation is more restrictive or more permissive, depending on the state. There is no ban on gamete donation and payment for the act is not explicitly prohibited. Some states allow both financial compensation for a surrogate mother and the existence of commercial surrogacy agencies (LUNA, 2002).

Jasanoff (2005) characterises the country's way of legislating as a "regime of rights" based on the individual right to choose, which is guided by the many contractual and individual forms that overlap and differ from state to state. The lack of specific regulations on assisted reproduction in the country would further favour this regime of rights.

In Germany, the laws are stricter and, for this reason, the impediments are greater than in other countries. The dissociation of genetic and gestational maternity is forbidden. Surrogate motherhood is forbidden and any woman who decides to donate her child is denied fertilisation. As for gamete donation, only semen donation is accepted, but only in cases of sterility in married couples.

France is characterised by its preoccupation with the ethical issues surrounding conceptive technologies, showing conservatism when dealing with the subject, which would result in a predisposition to develop so-called "reproductive tourism". In other words, the French have often contracted ART services in other countries, whose regulations are more flexible than in their country of origin (LUNA, 2002).

In 1994, the law regulating reproductive technologies was enacted in the country, which banned the use of surrogate pregnancies. The use of surplus embryos is only permitted with the authorisation of the two providers of the genetic material. French legislation interprets egg donation as the desire of the couple and the donor to establish parenthood with the woman who gives birth, based on the criterion of "the birth makes the mother". As there are no surrogacy contracts, the gestational mother, regardless of whether she has a genetic link, can keep the child if she so wishes, and it is debatable whether she is obliged to return the money received for the "service", in other words, surrogacy does not offer the slightest guarantee to the creators of this type of procreation that they will receive the desired baby (LUNA, 2002).

When the practice is effective, the surrogacy arrangement takes place with the father of the requesting couple recognising paternity from conception, while the gestational mother gives up her child for adoption and the woman of the couple adopts her husband's child. As far as gamete donation is concerned, the practice must be completely anonymous. Furthermore, it is not possible to use both donated gametes (LUNA, 2002; ALLEBRANDT, 2008).

In Brazil, human reproductive technologies have been provisionally standardised through Resolution 1.358/92 of the CFM (Federal Council of Medicine)[8] , through which ethical principles and norms have been adopted for the use of this medical speciality. The terms of the resolution were approved by the country's first bill, number 3638/93. Bill 2855/97 maintained the same content as the previous one. The next, No. 90/99, was the most open to discussions on the subject, with the aim of presenting justifications for establishing definitive legislation for the medical speciality in question.

According to researcher Fernanda Bittencourt Vieira, who studies the process of regulating conceptive technologies in Brazil, the main players represented in the

[8] A copy of the Resolution is attached.

debates on the latest bill were doctors, bioethicists, feminists, parliamentarians, legal experts and public prosecutors. A psychologist and a member of the LGBTT (Lesbian, Gay, Bisexual, Transvestite and Transsexual) movement also made occasional appearances. It was interesting to note that no users of assisted reproduction were present (VIEIRA, 2008).

According to the author, the discussions held within the scope of the Bills "are discourses that speak about and to a heterosexual, middle or upper class couple", because "The couple who cannot have biological children without the 'help' of technology is the discursive foundation of the assisted reproduction offer" (VIEIRA, 2008, p. 146-147). Currently, Bill No. 90/99 is being processed in the Chamber of Deputies under No. 1184/2003, and other Bills on the subject that were originally proposed in the Chamber have been added to it.

In these terms, Brazil has been characterised by a lack of debate on conceptive technologies. It is interesting to note that in 2000, the article *New reproductive technologies in Brazil: a debate awaiting regulation* was published by researchers Marilena Corrêa and Débora Diniz, which discussed the lack of debate in the field of assisted reproduction. Today, HTs are still waiting for definitive regulation. According to the researchers:

> In this regulatory process, at least three bills on "Assisted Human Reproduction" are currently underway in Brazil. All of them form a counterpoint to the 1992 CFM resolution, which is a normative reference to those bills. We didn't find a single new point to be observed, but only greater or lesser agreement or disagreement with the points raised in that inaugural 1992 text. Even on the issue of time and the availability of technologies that didn't exist in 1992, the bills make no progress (CORRÊA; DINIZ, 2000, p. 2).

The biggest discussion in the country on the subject of conceptive technologies dealt with the *Biosafety Law of* 2007, which authorised research into embryonic stem cells in surplus embryos from assisted reproduction treatments by the Supreme Court, when questions about the fate of embryos and the beginning of life were discussed. However, issues relating to: the practice of assisted reproduction , the need for specific legislation, as well as the control and supervision of clinics and semen banks, were not even mentioned.

As for the CFM Resolution, among its general principles, the document makes it clear that assisted reproduction plays an auxiliary role in solving human infertility problems, facilitating the process of procreation when other therapies have been ineffective or inefficient in solving the problem.

With regard to the gamete donation resource, the Resolution in question states the following:

IV - DONATION OF GAMETES OR PRE-EMBRYOS:

2 - Donors must not know the identity of recipients, and vice versa.

3 - The identity of gamete and pre-embryo donors and recipients must be kept confidential. In special situations, for medical reasons, information about donors can be provided exclusively to doctors, with the donor's civil identity being protected.

In order to comply with the recommendations in question, the parties involved in the donation process (donor, doctor responsible for the CT treatment and recipient) sign terms declaring their acceptance of the regulations. As mentioned above, the donor signs the document at the time of his selection by the semen bank. Later, at the stage when the treatment is about to be carried out, the doctor in charge

or the clinic to which it belongs provides a *consent form* for the recipient, which must include the signatures, with notarised signatures, of both parties (doctor and user) and two other witnesses. An original of the document is provided for both the professional and the client.

For around eighteen years, the aforementioned Resolution has provided guidelines for conceptual reproductive technologies. However, its permanence, to the detriment of a law drafted by the Law discipline, has generated controversy. With regard to the need to formulate specific legislation for the use of ART, opinions are divided. Among doctors, the need for regulation doesn't seem to occupy a privileged place in the debates, as they believe that the CFM Resolution in force is precise and sufficient to regulate these practices. This position was shared by the management of the semen bank surveyed and even by some legal professionals, such as judges and magistrates. For them, formulating a law is not a priority, and the request for it should come from medical professionals (ALLEBRANDT, 2007).

According to the testimony of a judge, provided for a survey that investigated the subject in Porto Alegre - RS, the formulation of a law is not a priority, and it is even premature to create legislation under current conditions, sharing the idea with other professionals interviewed that the law is always after the facts. For them:

> There are no rules on this, there are no rules in force in Brazil. These are all issues to be resolved. [...] From my point of view, I think it was a good thing that the code didn't say anything about this. Because it's far from being understood by us, imagine legislating on this. It's the kind of thing that you're going to legislate if there's not the slightest consensus, there's not the slightest

> understanding yet, is there? What is it, what does it entail, what are the consequences, where does it come from, where does it go? We don't know yet. So I think it's very premature to make legislation on this at the moment (ALLEBRANDT; MACEDO, 2007, p. 24).

In contrast to the position of the above subjects, some scholars emphasise the great need to regulate the use of reproductive technologies. Ferriani (2005) states that clinics are more concerned with debating freezing techniques than with the ethical aspects involved in freezing embryos. Guilhem (2000) points out that there is a lack of transparency regarding the practices carried out by assisted reproduction clinics. The author reports a case that occurred at the Maternal and Child Hospital in Brasilia, where a woman had five embryos implanted at once, whereas the recommendation expressed in current Brazilian regulations is a maximum of three per attempt.

As a result of the large number of embryos implanted, the babies were born with serious health problems, requiring hospitalisation in a neonatal intensive care unit (ICU) for two months. During this period, one of them died and, of the remaining four, three have cerebral palsy. Based on this example, the author emphasises the need for legislation on this issue (ALLEBRANDT; MACEDO, 2007, p. 24).

Opposing the above-mentioned position of doctors, judges and magistrates, lawyers Moura and Cenedeze (2001) share the idea of researcher Guilhem (2000) that there is a need to draw up a specific law for the practice, based primarily on hierarchy and legislative dissonance. For them, because a resolution is a purely normative act that, as a rule, concerns administrative or regulatory issues of the institution that issued it, the document issued by the CFM does not have the competence to regulate a medical practice that is so complex and has such relevant medical, ethical, social, cultural and religious implications that are still so little known.

The authors specifically analyse heterologous assisted reproduction, which would be in conflict with the Brazilian Federal Constitution and the Statute of the Child and Adolescent, with regard to the right to life, human dignity and the recognition of the state of filiation.

> (...) Within this theme, we will finally turn our attention to a new reality in genetic engineering: semen banks. If the rule for this system is to hide the identification of the donors or sellers of the material used, how would this affect the constitutional principles of the right to life, human dignity and the recognition of the state of filiation as a very personal, unavailable and imprescriptible right, as laid down in the Statute of the Child and Adolescent [ECA - Law 8.069/90]? (MOURA; CENEDEZE, 2001, p. 126).

In line with the above, the legal sphere does not seem to be able to provide satisfactory answers to the problems that have arisen as a result of conceptive technologies at the present time and, with regard to conception with anonymous semen donation, the great controversy seems to be over the secrecy of the donor's identity, due to the fact that it harms the right to inheritance and its fundamental guarantees: the right to paternity investigation, the right to inheritance, alimony and the right to nationality, as well as concealing the matrimonial impediments provided for in article 183, of the Brazilian Civil Code.

> According to paragraph 6 of article 227 of the Federal Constitution, "(...) children, whether or not born of wedlock, or by adoption, shall have the same rights and qualifications, and any discriminatory designations relating to filiation shall be prohibited." (MOURA; CENEDEZE, 2001, p. 130).

Also, according to the researchers, only constitutional precepts can provide satisfactory answers to the legal gap between insemination and gamete donation,

> [...] whether now, while the relevant regulations have not been published, or once they have been drawn up and are in force, the issue of genetic manipulation must be calibrated at all times in the light of constitutional principles - the only way to ensure that the paths of progress are opened up within the fundamental frameworks freely established by society. (FERRAS apud MOURA; CENEDEZE, 2001, p. 126-127).

Although some legal professionals want to transfer to the medical sphere the right and duty to legislate on a speciality governed by the profession, there is a legislative hierarchy and the Federal Constitution is sovereign, to which every act and every Brazilian citizen must submit. In this sense, although at the moment there are more open questions than solutions to them, it can be said that, legally, "[...] the act issued by the CFM is in total disagreement not only with our ordinary legislation, but also with express constitutional provisions". (MOURA; CENEDEZE, 2001, p. 130).

It is interesting to note that the Resolution governing the practice was produced by a Professional Council belonging to the medical profession, a profession that both produces the technologies dealt with here and is produced by them. This seems to be part of the important processes of medicalisation of different aspects of life that in the past turned obstetrics into a profession, as well as pregnancy and everything that comes from it, including technology, into "medicalisable" and "pathologisable" phenomena, as a result of disciplinary power: subjectivising and normatising. (CORRÊA, 2001; TESSER, 2006).

According to information provided by the São Paulo semen bank, the first birth from semen donation took place just sixteen years ago and, in most cases, couples seem to opt for absolute secrecy, even among their family and friends. However, the "veil" being drawn over the biological origins of these children is no guarantee of their infallibility. Taking the United States as a reference, there have been frequent cases in which, in order to obtain access to information about the identity of gamete donors, there are alternative ways of finding these individuals who are represented in the speeches of their "children" as the "invisible/hidden side" or the "missing link". The protagonist of numerous stories in The New *York Times* is the website "donor sibling registry"[9] , created by Wendy Kraemer, the mother of a son of an anonymous semen donor who wanted to meet his biological "father". As a result, the boy ended up finding his siblings and making it possible for others to do the same (ALLEBRANDT, 2008).

It's possible that the maturing of these Brazilian children, their experiences and life within the "new families" will lead to the emergence of facts that will favour alternative ways of getting closer to the "missing link", as was the case with Wendy Kraemer. It may also be that these events will lead to demands for more coherent and fair guidelines from the law in relation to hetero-orthogamous assisted reproduction practices, especially here in Brazil, where decision-making power reigns in the hands of a small group, misinformation on the part of users and governmental evasion. Alternatively, it is likely that the same facts will lead to a more involved questioning of the social effects of conception with gamete donation.

[9] http://www.donor sibling registry.com.

CHAPTER 2

SOCIAL IMPLICATIONS OF ASSISTED REPRODUCTION PRACTICES

I decided to start this chapter with an account of an experience with motherhood through the "hands" of technology, because the material "speaks for itself" and will be presented throughout these pages. The interviewee's story highlights some of the main issues surrounding artificial procreation today. Various phenomena are interwoven in this scenario: the desire for children, which is a social norm; the social medicalisation of human reproduction, translated into a scheme for regulating individuals, in which the specialist is the holder of power and infertility is the target of medical correction, carried out by means of its technological instruments; the social effects produced by the results of the techniques and their consequences for subjectivity, which can be drastic, and which have commonly been experienced in solitude.

The case of Alíscia Baensi

Aliscia Baensi[10] , forty years old, a middle-class teacher living in the north of Rio de Janeiro, divorced for four years, mother of six-year-old Luma, became pregnant through artificial insemination with anonymous semen donation because Pedro, to whom she had been married for ten years, was sterile. After years of trying, they went to a specialist who recommended the treatment as the best for the couple, due to its simplicity and low cost. They used all their savings to try to conceive. At that time, in 2002, around $5,000.00 (five thousand dollars) was spent on consultations, medication for hormonal hyperstimulation, tests and procedures, and eighteen months later they were successful. The truth about the couple's experience was concealed from their social relationships in order to preserve their privacy and contribute to the "naturalness" of reproduction.

However, the birth of their daughter brought deep conflicts for Alíscia and Pedro, both internal and familial. He felt on the margins of the mother-baby relationship, suffering from the lack of biogenetic affinity and phenotypic similarity with the child, which was reinforced by external comments. She felt lonely and guilty for having wanted to experience pregnancy, the main justification for her choice. Two years later, Pedro decided to separate and move to another state, and since then he has had little contact

[10] All first names mentioned in this thesis are fictitious.

with the two of them. Alíscia was able to establish a satisfactory bond with Luma, but has irreparable scars from the effects that the experience with assisted reproduction had on her life. In her opinion, there is still no room in society for these new families, which come to exist in a world hidden from the "real world", which doctors in the field should warn about, just as they inform their patients about techniques and values. According to Alíscia: "I only realised that the physical resemblance to the donor wasn't *going to* turn Luma into Pedro's daughter after she was born, and then it was too late. Doctors should have informed us of the possibility of these conflicts. It seems that only the technique has evolved, but the human side of this medicine doesn't exist. At least it didn't for my family."[11] .

* * *

The subject of assisted human reproduction has provoked a variety of discourses in academic circles, based on the notions of nature and culture, from which the boundary between the biological and the socially constructed is constantly rewritten.

To the discourse of the maternal instinct, reproductive technologies have associated the "desire for children", which in turn has opened up new demands for the right to choose "how to have children", which in turn has opened up a range of options for this choice: *in vitro* fertilisation, "surrogacy", insemination with gamete donation, and even the possibility of using an artificial womb.

The insertion of this speciality into society has led to changes in people's reproductive behaviour, as it breaks down the sex/reproduction dyad with its treatments, breaks the reproduction/gestation *continuum* with surrogate pregnancies, makes it possible to choose the child you want to have through pre-implantation diagnosis (PID), as well as exercising a kind of control over sex and human reproduction.

ART and its various arrangements aimed at achieving pregnancy have realised ideals of life, but they have also produced consequences in various areas, some of which are not yet foreseeable. The debates that have been taking place in academic circles, ethics and bioethics address issues such as: the fate of supernumerary embryos (freezing, research, disposal, donation), the aspects of eugenics and racial and sexual discrimination

[11] This story is the result of an interview the protagonist gave me in July 2009. A mutual friend of both of us mentioned my research during a conversation with Alíscia, which sparked her interest in sharing her experience with someone who, according to her judgement, would be able to understand her and at the same time contribute to the research. The material is digitally recorded.

reinforced by the practice, as well as the conflicts that are being generated at the level of the family, filiation, sexuality, subjectivity, etc? which are being governed by the phenomenon of social medicalisation, which imposes a norm of the desire for descent (SALÉM, 1995; SCAVONE, 1998; CORRÊA, 2001; TAMANINI, 2003; COSTA, 2004; ALLEMBRANDT, 2008). This chapter will address some of these effects, focusing on the practice of using donated gametes.

2.1 Social medicalisation and the desire for offspring

> It's common to dream, I know, when evening comes.
> Well, I've had a dream too, and it's so beautiful.
> I see a cradle and I'm leaning over it, crying.
> And so, crying, I cherish the child I want to have.
> Sleep, my little one, sleep because life is coming.
> Your father is very lonely with all the love he has [...].
>
> When life finally wants to take me for all that it has given me.
> To feel his beard brushing against me in his last kiss.
> And when I also felt your hand sealing my gaze from your eyes.
> Listening to her voice lulling me into a goodbye song.
> Sleep, my father, without a care, sleep that evening.
> Your son daydreams about the son he wants to have.
>
> Music:
> The son I want to have.
> (TOQUINHO and VINÍCIUS DE MORAES, 1975).

According to anthropological studies, it cannot be said that interest in the issue of procreation is current and restricted to the society to which we belong. "The question of palliatives for sterility, which interests us so much today, has always been a concern of all societies" (HÉRITIER, 2000, p. 99), since the desire for children and offspring is found in most human groups. For the author, "(...) it seems to be more a desire for offspring and a desire for fulfilment than a desire for children, and more a need to fulfil a duty to oneself and to the community than a claim to the right to possess." (HÉRITIER, 2000, p. 99) (HÉRITIER, 2000, p. 103). Procreation would then be almost a duty for all individuals and not fulfilling it would be a "crime against oneself".

same, here and hereafter", as can be exemplified by the case of the Samo. [12] (HÉRITIER, 2000, p. 104). "Desire and duty of descent. Not to pass on one's life is to break a chain in which no one *is the* ultimate end and is, on the other hand, to forbid oneself access to the *status of* ancestor". (HÉRITIER, 2000, p.103).

[12] In the case of the Samo, a community located in Burkina Faso, an African country, women who die without procreating and whose destiny has not been fulfilled are seen as jealous and go on to attack the living, bringing them unhappiness. A visceral discontent makes them demons of such a dangerous nature that even the other demons move out of their way.

The issue of infertility is resolved in different ways in different cultural contexts, such as a form of marriage among the Nuer, tribes of pastoralists in Sudan, located on the African continent, which takes place between two women as a way of "reversing" the inability to procreate.

> This is a situation in which a woman who is proven to be sterile takes up her original lineage to produce offspring. She becomes a man and can marry another woman. Through access to her brothers' jointly owned property, to which she is now entitled, she enters into marriage using the usual dowry system. The wife serves her husband and works for his benefit. The children - the result of the wife's sexual relations with a man from outside the community, often from another ethnic group or a prisoner - recognise the husband-wife as their father and call her that [...] (HEILBORN, 1991, p. 32).

In this sense, there seems to be an identifiable concern in almost every human society to solve the problem of childlessness, both biologically and socially, implying more or less visible arrangements between individuals of both sexes, indicating at the same time that sterility has always been socially frowned upon and repudiated as an unfortunate condition. It is in this context that technological advances in the medical field are inserted, aiming to "solve" the "problem" of infertility.

Reproductive technologies are an exercise in the medicalisation of childlessness, which presupposes "(...) a norm - of motherhood and/or reproduction - whose deviation would be legitimately corrected by means of technological intervention proposals that result in test tube babies." (CORRÊA, 2001, p. 24), being identified as the apex of the process of social medicalisation of sexuality and reproduction, with social normalisation as its function.

The phenomenon of social medicalisation produces a centralisation and control in the actions and heteronomous interpretations of biomedicine over subjects, culturally transforming populations as a result of the decline in their ability to cope autonomously with most of their illnesses and daily pains, leading to abusive and counterproductive consumption of these services, generating excessive dependence and alienation. Subjects, submitted to the discourses of medical normalisation, end up being referred to the intervention of some specialised practice (TESSER, 2006).

Medicalisation encompasses various phenomena and was widely used in studies analysing and criticising medical consumption in the 1960s. Thus, the term social medicalisation refers, on the one hand, to the way in which continuous technological evolution has modified medical practice, through innovations in the field of diagnostic and therapeutic methods, the pharmaceutical industry, medical equipment, etc. The process of social medicalisation also redescribes physiological aspects such as pregnancy, childbirth, menopause, ageing, as well as deviant social behaviour: unsuitability for work, drug use, alcoholism, among others (CORRÊA, 2001).

These descriptions have an effect on medical consumption and on the production of knowledge by medicine and common social representations, which are subjected to discursive medical normalisation and end up being referred to the intervention of some specialised practice. Finally, social medicalisation is also used to refer to the game of interests involved in the very production of medical acts, which implies an expansion of profits in the commercialisation of services, equipment and products, particularly associated with technological proliferation (TAMANINI, 2003).

Reproductive technologies are part of a field marked by complexity, control, the power of science and technology over society, the practice of *experimentation* and their low *performance, which is* generally hidden. Corrêa (2001, p. 74) chose the technique of *in vitro* fertilisation as an example and found that the way in which conceptive technologies are disseminated, by various professionals (doctors, biologists, psychologists or journalists), creates "the illusion of simple and immediate access to a baby, provided by IVF and generated by the demand of an individual or couple", which would place the speciality between a "science of *experts"* and common knowledge, which would characterise it as a *vade mecum*[13] *science,* but which, on the other hand, would be a science that omits details and controversies through stylistic artifice, leaving information about stages, the professional required, the destination of the material collected, efficacy, etc. in the shadows., especially controversies within the scientific milieu itself about technical details, which is specific to the medical school itself, because it rules out dilemmas, scientific vulgarisation or lay dissemination (ARKSEY apud CORRÊA, 2001).

Taking the case of Alíscia Baensi, which introduced this chapter, as a point of support, the assisted reproduction technique, which was presented to the interviewee as simple and without risks for the woman, is actually part of a field where there is strict control of the details of each stage and the insemination process is far from simple, as it involves: female hormonal hyperstimulation, which is carried out by medication on the part of the woman; maturation of the ovarian follicles, which is monitored and assessed according to their morphological characteristics by means of various ultrasounds, as well

---

[13] *Vade-mecum* is a Latin expression meaning "come with me", and today it is used to indicate a book, or a collection of texts on a particular subject or area of science, which are condensed or simplified by its "Organiser". Available at http://shoppingdosaber.com.br. Consulted on 24/11/2008, at 19:34 hs.

as laboratory tests; preparation of the spermatozoa; fertilisation of the egg; the pregnancy phase, which must also be pharmacologically maintained. Finally, the birth.

For these steps to be completed satisfactorily, AR centres need to have high-tech equipment, specialised culture articles, materials for toxicity tests on containers and culture media, laboratory facilities capable of examining semen, with equipment for handling gametes and embryos and for hormone assessment (radioimmunoassay), ultrasound machines and facilities for minor surgical interventions. As for the professional staff, they are highly qualified in a variety of areas, such as: a gynaecologist with training in sterility and reproductive endocrinology, an ultrasonographer, a biologist with experience in clinical embryology and tissue culture; laboratory technicians with experience in the area, a nurse to monitor the procedures and also social and/or psychological staff, whose presence during the execution of the techniques is required by the Ethics Committees, especially in first world countries (CORRÊA, 2001, p. 76), which is not the rule in Brazil.

As a result, heavy demands are placed on the users of these technologies, when they are given huge responsibilities for the treatment and a real job, with routine tasks, use of medication, precisely scheduled doctor and laboratory visits. Exposure to these treatments presents a series of risks for women, linked to high doses of hormones, anaesthesia for punctures (in the case of IVF treatment), risks of various infections, multiple pregnancies, which add up to enormous physical and emotional strain. This whole reality is intensified by the fact that the efficiency of reproductive procedures is unsafe and *underperforming*, despite media and professional reports to the contrary. The quote below illustrates this:

> [...] until the 1990s, the success of *in vitro* fertilisation techniques (determined as birth per stimulated cycle) in France and the United States , two of the main producers of this technology worldwide, did not exceed 13% of all attempts. Among the main problems in assessing the true success of IVF are the lack of uniformity in the criteria used and the omission of the source of information on data such as hormonal hyperstimulation - the phase that precedes oocyte puncture and actually corresponds to the start of IVF treatment [...] (CORRÊA, 2001, p. 94).

As for the cost of HTs, contrary to what was mentioned in the situation of interviewee Alíscia Baensi, "(...) In addition to the time spent by the people involved, especially the woman, and all the wear and tear already described, treatment using assisted reproduction techniques has a very high financial cost". (CORRÊA, p. 90).

Looking for an estimate and comparison of the cost of reproductive treatment, based on IVF, each attempt would cost an average of three thousand dollars in France, between three and six thousand dollars in the US, and between three and five thousand dollars in Brazil. Considering that failure rates are over 80 per cent, a pregnancy - which does not mean a guaranteed birth - could cost around twenty thousand dollars at the end of the 1980s (MARCUS-STEIFF apud CORRÊA, 2001, p. 90).

It's important to point out that, in general, treatments with CRTs are paid for by the patient themselves, which varies between nations. Taking into account data from nine years ago, in some European countries, such as France, these costs are usually financed predominantly by social insurance systems. When they are carried out by the private sector, they generally correspond to those cases for which the use of assisted reproduction is not provided for by law, or accepted in bioethical recommendations: those of single people, homosexuals and menopausal women. Germany has seen a trend towards cutting funding for the technology. In Australia, IVFs are financed by public funds, but have been cut back due to poor results. In the USA, as in Brazil, the costs are borne predominantly by the clients (CORRÊA, 2001).

The hierarchical positions occupied by the specialist and the patient are also an important aspect of assisted reproduction, which is in line with the phenomenon of social medicalisation. It can be seen that the doctor-patient relationship is based on a type of verticality, in which decision-making power is centralised in the hands of the professional, whose interests are always more focused on technical issues (in some cases, financial issues), in other words, on choosing the technique and conducting the treatment for the purpose of pregnancy. In this sense, we are led to ask whether human reproductive technologies are at the service of the requesting patient or another type of interest. What's more, users of these technologies aren't usually given proper guidance by professionals on the pros and cons of treatment with HTs, so that they can decide on their reproductive destiny, or perhaps this type of decision is also in the hands of the specialist, who holds the power that comes from knowledge, science and technology.

Novaes and Salem (1995) analyse reproductive technologies in terms of the medicalisation of reproduction, arguing that these techniques often promote the transfer of reproductive decisions from the woman or couple to doctors.

According to Corrêa,

> The "interest of the patient" which, as an ideal, may have guided and justified medicine in its progress, is becoming increasingly difficult to define. The current forms of organisation of medicine and the complexity of the technology associated with them greatly complicate what can be medically delimited as an *interest* in healing or well-being and, in many cases, remove or deepen the alienation of ordinary people from decision-making regarding their own bodies, their well-being and, ultimately, the fate of their lives (CORRÊA, 2001, p. 25).

In addition to the situations discussed here, reproductive technologies also have a significant impact on the sphere of family, kinship, sex and gender, promoting a re-signification of the notions we have built up in this regard. This theme will be presented below.

2.2 **Deconstructing notions, or today's new old families**

Socio-anthropological studies on the family and kinship have intensified with the historical transformations that have been taking place. Advances in the field of medicine and its links with reproductive technologies represent one of these changes (CABRAL, 2005). According to studies on the subject, the family ties established in contemporary times are based on blood ties and, paradoxically, the ideal of choice. It is important to emphasise that these characteristics are not universal. In other groups, the establishment of kinship is not always seen as a necessary consequence of the biological, or of a union based on love.

The Western model, which emphasises biological ties, is evident in law and has Roman origins, enshrining the formula of the Napoleonic Code of 1804 for the presumption of paternity. In other words, paternity is recognised as legitimate by proving the marriage of the presumed father to the child's mother, and maternity is taken for granted once the birth has been proven. Thus, the relationship of paternity and maternity rights must coincide with the "biological truth". Current legal interpretations of this type of kinship point out that individual will is the necessary complement to the biological bond, emphasising the importance of "lived filiation". (LEITE, 1995).

> According to the Brazilian Civil Code of 1916, the concept of a legally recognised family was based on the elements of consanguinity and formal marriage. However, these elements are now considered insufficient for recognising family relationships that presuppose affection, function and not just genetic correspondence. For the field of law, this possibility is extremely new, as until then it recognised genetic coincidence as the primary attribute for the conceptions of maternity and paternity [...] (SILVA; LOPES, 2008, p. 3).

This legal description of the establishment of kinship relations in the West coincides with Schneider's (1968 apud LUNA, 2002) analysis of American kinship symbolism, which highlights two basic aspects: blood ties, understood and updated by scientific language as ties of biogenetic substance (DNA). The second aspect is the code of conduct, which consists of the recognition of ties based on the behaviour of relatives. According to Leite (1995), blood ties would be the real foundation of kinship, considered irreversible, the "biological truth", while the code of conduct would be a constructed or revocable aspect.

Western kinship is made up of relationships based on procreation and the provision of care for offspring, prioritising relationships and the formation of a matrix of relationships. The idea of family, on the other hand, is associated with the institutional aspect. Thus, each person would belong to a kinship constellation, justifying the notions of kinship relations as something of the private order in relation to society, which would also reinforce the need for the transmission of biological characteristics (LUNA, 2007).

Anthropologist Claudia Fonseca also analyses contemporary families based on two concomitant and contradictory principles, which are congruent with those highlighted by Schneider and Leite. The first refers to the notion of the family based on biological factors, or the genetic code determining family belonging, and the second refers to the notion of the *man-made* family, whose emphasis centres on the ideal of choice, love and happiness.

> Historians describe how, especially since the Industrial Revolution, love has come to be seen as a fundamental factor in family life. Children, seen in pre-modern times as labour for the family business, security in old age or a means of perpetuating the lineage, came to have a primarily affective value. In the same way, romantic love characterises the ideal marriage, dictating the need for a "free choice" of spouse. Here the central value is no longer the lineage or the family name, to be protected at any cost (by sacrificing certain members when necessary), but the happiness of the individuals (FONSECA, 2002, p. 273).

According to the author, the current emphasis on choice and affection would also allow for the legitimisation and proliferation of previously unaccepted family forms, such as adoptive filiation, same-sex relationships and recomposed families, which, combined with historical factors, transform family life into a porous space, permeated by forces (fluctuations in the job market, the inclusion of women in this market, home financing policies, political persecution, nationality laws...) and relationships (with grandparents, nannies...) that extend far beyond the domestic unit.) and relationships (with grandparents, nannies, schools...) that extend far beyond the domestic unit. Added to these families are those built through reproductive technologies and their countless kinship arrangements, forming what the researcher calls "families on the move". (FONSECA, 2007). On the other hand, these same families also reinforce the value placed on ties by consanguinity.

Borlot and Trindade (2004) carried out a study with infertile couples who had undergone treatment with reproductive technologies and had been unsuccessful. The researchers analysed the couples' lives from the moment infertility was diagnosed, in order to identify what social representations they had of a biological child. The results obtained indicate that these social representations are related to the desire for consanguineous descent as a continuation of the paternal and maternal families, the importance of pregnancy, the desire to have a child with physical similarities to the parents and social pressure, which greatly influences the couple's decisions.

Naara Luna (2002) conducted interviews with women who were undergoing treatment to become pregnant in private assisted reproduction clinics, in order to investigate the group's notions of kinship and consanguinity. According to the researcher's analyses, blood articulates both the order of nature and the order of culture. This substance seems to transmit physical and moral characteristics, forming the body and character (ABREU FILHO, 1982). In this sense, the individual is explained by reference to their consanguineous relatives, in other words, as a result of this transmission of attributes, the person is born morally constituted, representative of a family, of a tradition.

In this sense, kinship is revealed as a language of belonging. There is a desire for a communion of substance with children, which is revealed in the testimony of one interviewee. In her opposition to adoption, Rosilda speaks of the idealised biological child as "my flesh", "my blood", producing a contrast between her own child and the child of another. It's interesting to note that although blood ties can be interpreted in terms of a biogenetic connection (SCHNEIDER apud LUNA, 2004, p. 237), referring to a person's physical characteristics, the informants who expressed fear of adoption mentioned temperament and social traits more often. The following quotes illustrate this:

> Rosilda says: "If I were to adopt, I'd want a newborn. Big ones, three or four years old, I don't want, because they're already rebellious". Mariana continues: "Because, if the child has a problem, you'll say: well, that's not my child. It came from the blood... I don't know whose blood that is? Whose blood? This bad temper." (LUNA, 2004, p. 130).

Based on Naara Luna's analyses, the family and kinship relationships arising from reproductive technologies break with the chain of events that we have traditionally experienced, which links marriage, sexual intercourse, pregnancy, childbirth and motherhood. For these relationships to be successful, it is necessary to employ the principles of the American ideology of kinship, maintained in the family and in biogenetics. Maternity and paternity are reconceptualised as social and biological, with the intention of the couple or the individual being the reason for the baby's conception (LUNA, 2002). Let's look at the following quote:

> The technologies of procreation are means of obtaining children, generally by circumventing situations of sterility. Comparing the representations of sterility in the ethnographic accounts of different societies, Héritier (1984) observes that the behavioural faults sanctioned by sterility involve the crossing of generations, the crossing of bloods and the crossing of genders. These are acts of transgression that disrupt the cosmic order and its balance. Life is transmitted according to the order of generations: parents stop procreating when their children are married. The fusion of substances in marriage is regulated, with a ban on consanguineous unions and adultery. Finally, contamination between the male and female genders is avoided in the practices of homosexuality, self-sexuality (masturbation), and between other genders that must be kept separate (incestuous relations, with animals, or with beings from beyond). This disruption of the cosmic order concerns the rules of kinship. The technologies of conception open up space for such ruptures when women after the age of menopause give birth, daughters donate eggs for their mothers to become pregnant, mothers give up their wombs to receive the embryos formed with gametes from their sons and daughters-in-law, homosexual couples make children, ovarian and testicular tissues are cultivated in host animals (Luna, 2001b, 2002[a]). The technical possibility of mixing generations, mixing blood and genders is created through the use of assisted reproduction (LUNA, 2007, p. 181).

The improvements to nature brought about by reproductive techniques are considered acceptable, as long as the changes are in line with the principles of nature (HIRSCH, 1999), because, according to Salem (1995), the legitimacy of kinship relationships engendered through reproductive technologies presupposes their similarity and proximity to biologically or genetically given relationships, which constitutes an affirmation of the natural order (nature) as the moral order par excellence.

With regard to kinship, reproductive technologies can act in three ways: (1) reinforcing the importance given to the biological aspect of reproduction; (2) interfering in what is considered "biological truth", creating a reality in which both the genetic mother and father can be different from the social father and mother or even the gestational mother, (3) reinforcing the intentional aspect of kinship (SALEM, 1995).

Researchers have dedicated themselves to studying the reconfigurations of family and kinship as a result of the insertion of reproductive technologies into human life. Based on an investigation comparing surrogate motherhood and egg donation, Cussins (1998) argues against the existence of a fixed and unique natural basis for the relevant categories of kinship. His thesis is that there are elements that are considered relevant (opaque) to kinship and those that are irrelevant (transparent) and that these are distributed in different ways in each procedure.

The stages in the development of a pregnancy that generate kinship are called *opaque*: genetics, socio-economic factors (who pays for the treatment), legal factors (who owns the gametes and embryos) and family factors (whose partner is the sperm supplier, or who will take responsibility for the child). The *transparent* stage contributes to the process, but is not configured in the web of kinship. In this way, undesirable links are erased (transparent) and appropriate ones emphasised (opaque). The following situations demonstrate how undesirable links can be erased and appropriate ones made opaque. In the experience in which a woman serves as a surrogate for her brother, the bond formed between one and the other must be erased (transparent), in order to emphasise that the gametes of the two did not unite. In the gestational surrogacy experience, the surrogate mother must become irrelevant as to the kinship of the baby after its birth (transparent). The kinship of a surrogate mother becomes relevant (opaque) because she is married to the baby's genetic father (opaque), because she has the secret of her daughter being the egg donor (transparent) and because she can afford (opaque) a surrogate (transparent). Opaque and transparent links must be separated to determine who is related to whom.

According to the researcher's analyses, the cultural is not simply based on the natural, but the natural gains explanatory power by being linked to culturally relevant categories. Phenomena considered natural are read as socialised: pregnancy is equated with caring for a child. Genetics can also be socialised in the search for egg donors of the same ethnic origin as the recipient. On the other hand, community practices to help with childcare are naturalised when looking for a donor in that environment. Semen donation and egg donation form different configurations of kinship.

According to Marylin Strathern (1995a), in the face of reproductive technologies, "a new field of kinship relations has partially displaced the family as an arena in which people work out the implications of their reproductive practices". (STRATHERN, 1995a, p. 347). For the author, who takes the "natural fact" as the foundation of Euro-American perceptions (kinship is seen as comprising both social and natural elements), the new visions of the process do not do away with the family, but risk producing "more kinship, less relations", i.e. the identification of genetic connections without necessarily the social relations that have normally defined "kin".

The researcher points to the need to associate kinship and bilateral parenting, since parenting is linked to the notion of having identifiable parents who are equal in the sense of their genetic contribution. However, in the case of gamete donation, these parents will be unequal in terms of the roles they play, which would unbalance the complex equation between kinship and parenthood. Therefore, in the case of the use of assisted reproduction, there must be a negotiation about what a family is or from what assumptions it is built.

One proposal that has been widely accepted in academic circles is that of Janet Carsten, in her work *Cultures of Relatedness*, where the author moves away from the discussion about the opposition between biological and social. Carsten proposes a change in vocabulary: the use of the term 'connectedness' *reilatednsssy'Qxri* opposition or alongside kinship to signal an opening up to indigenous languages of connectedness". (CARSTEN, 2000, p. 4). The collection she has organised presents ethnographic examples of contemporary situations in China, Alaska, Madagascar and England (among others) in order to understand which symbols - apart from blood, semen and breast milk - refer to "shared *substance*" and which create the kind of deep and lasting relationship normally associated with the kinship sphere.

The criteria used for conceptive technologies and the way this medical speciality is legislated in various countries[14] reflect the tendency to make "natural" filiation the model for artificial procreation. It so happens that, even if various arrangements are made with the aim of achieving symmetry between assisted reproduction and natural reproduction, even if artificial procreation seeks to adapt to the socially accepted model of family and kinship, prioritising phenotypic similarity , based on the regulations for assisted reproduction, the family formed by these technologies is not the same as the traditional nuclear family model, especially if gametes from third parties are used.

In order for the first type of family to "appear" to resemble the second, the truth about its origins needs to be hidden, often from the child themselves, as well as from their closest family and friends. Everything indicates that this is the path commonly chosen by the creators of this type of reproduction. However, the concealment of a life situation does not mean its disappearance or non-existence, nor does it transform the family formed by assisted reproduction into a "traditional" family.

In a comparison between donation and adoption, Claudia Fonseca states that:

> [...] in the current legal system, there is a desire to "imitate nature" or copy a "normal" family - which, according to the hegemonic and traditional model, is made up of the "nucleus": father, mother and child. In this way, there is no room for other mums and dads. If they do exist - as in the case of adoption or heterologous donation - they must be kept out of the picture in order to maintain the illusion of a "natural" family. (FONSECA apud ALLEBRANDT, 2008, p. 80).

There is evidence that the families "produced" by reproductive technologies have not yet been satisfactorily integrated into society. It can be seen that both the actors and the RA scene are immersed in controversy, confusion, doubts, fears and silence, and this reality does not vary between countries, where medical societies and ethics

[14] The subject was covered in section 2.3

committees have taken different positions in the face of the new issues that have arisen. Many situations are still received by others with perplexity; the users of these technologies themselves often act in such a way as to hide the true processes of their children's generation, often from their own children, and the professionals responsible for the treatments often act in such a way as to protect their patients from the outside world, possibly more out of their own interests than those of the patient.

On the other side are the co-producers of reproduction (donors, gamete donors and surrogate mothers) who are more submerged in anonymity, silenced and powerless than the other two vertices of the artificial procreation triangle: idealising parents and doctors. They are all protected from contact and dialogue by a *consent form* that "guarantees" (or imposes) anonymity, as if hiding the truth could be the truth, which is fact and is there in the experience of events and in the experience of emotions. If these families are "kept out of the picture in order to maintain the illusion of a 'natural' family", it is clear that they are not "natural", since illusion is synonymous with "deception of the senses or mind, which causes one to take one thing for another, to misinterpret a fact or sensation" (DICIONÁRIO AURÉLIO *ONLINE).*

Within families that use reproductive technologies, there are likely to be conflicts, doubts and guilt, so the question arises: what happens when users of assisted reproduction realise their dream of a "biological child"? What kind of experiences have families who have used reproductive technologies had and do they still have today? How do the individuals involved in this type of procreation build bonds of kinship with the idealised baby? How do these individuals deal with the "presence" of the anonymous donor within the family? What quality of feelings inhabits the individual who has been excluded from the genetic make-up of the conceived child and, on the other hand, how does the individual who is a biological part of this child with the donor feel, with their partner left out? How does the relationship between the couple develop after the experience with assisted reproduction? How do single and menopausal women and same-sex couples who have used heterologous assisted reproduction fit into this context? How does the child itself fit in and develop in the family environment? Furthermore, how are the problems regarding the child's origins resolved?

Marilena Corrêa presents a study conducted by a psychoanalyst in an IVF service in France, which involved thirty-three mother-child pairs. Fifteen children born through egg donation were compared with two other groups, one of children born to infertile mothers who became pregnant after ovarian stimulation alone and the other through natural procreation. Since pregnancy with egg donation is an aspect that dissociates the mother's biological identity into: an ovarian mother (the genetic one) and a uterine mother, the authors, who interviewed and visited the research participants at home at 9 (nine) and 18 (eighteen) months, and then at 3 (three) years after the birth, found that

> (...) the genetic aspect of the oocyte is forgotten by the quality of the relational and physiological mother-child exchanges that take place throughout pregnancy. Finally, the birth has just sealed, at the level of the body, the intimate conviction that this child is very much yours. The anonymity of the donor seems to allow the mother-to-be to more easily project her personal history and her own identificatory models onto the child (RAOUL- DUVAL et al. apud CORRÊA, 2001, p. 181).

The results of another study carried out at the French network of semen banks (CECOS) in 1996 point to differences in relation to the data obtained in the research with mothers of children born with donated eggs (MANUEL apud CORRÊA, 2001). In the research in question, 96 (ninety-six) interviews were carried out with parents of children born through artificial insemination with a donor, when their children were three, eighteen and thirty-six months old, and with another thirty-four people who had undergone conservative treatments for infertility. The aim of the study was to analyse concerns about the similarity between parents and children in cases of donated reproductive material.

Some individuals (9 per cent) commented on the reaction of their immediate social environment. Regardless of the positive or negative correlation related to the similarity between father and son, these comments were felt to be painful because they were perceived by the couple as a reference to their transgression of cultural and social norms (MANUEL apud CORRÊA, 2001, p. 186). In addition, they provoked feelings of distrust among those couples who had chosen to confide in friends and/or relatives about donating gametes for artificial insemination. Even in the absence of comments, the researcher witnessed cases of depressed men who suffered from the non-similarity between them and the child, always referring to a specific physical characteristic (the blue eyes...)". There was even the case of the development of a delusional conviction in a man (who had followed the rules of anonymity and secrecy) who said: "Everyone knows, everyone doubts that this child is mine." (MANUEL apud CORRÊA, 2001, p. 186).

A study carried out in France points to an ambiguity identified among parents about revealing the truth about their child's origin to their child. The anonymity of the egg donors was valued by the participants, but few wanted to keep the way the child was conceived a secret. However, revealing their biological origin is a source of uncertainty and conflict, fearing a claim by the child to know their biological mother (RAOUL-DUVAL et al. apud CORRÊA, 2001).

Maria Consuêlo Passos, who studies the same-sex family, comments on some of the questions raised. Although she focuses on the homosexual family, her reflections can be transposed to other groups (infertile couples and celibate women), who will always have a third person mediating the "production" of children. For the researcher,

> (...) in all these family compositions there is the presence of a third party, mediating the desire to conceive a child. Ultimately, the couple depends on a third party to realise their project. This other, who will remain in the family's imagination and with whom the parents have to live, interferes in the formation of emotional ties with their children in different ways, depending on how it is assimilated/elaborated by the parents. Sometimes, the imaginary other takes the form of a figure that overlaps with the parents. At other times, it appears as an enigmatic shadow that accompanies and disturbs the children's recognition, and it can also be assimilated as an element without which filiation would not exist (PASSOS, 2005, p. 35).

In other words, the family relationships established through the anonymous donation of genetic material would be inserted in a context where the possibilities of experiencing conflicts seem to be quite significant. However, these bonds can be built in harmony. To this end, I believe it is necessary to transcend certain social rules so that the "presence of the anonymous donor can be assimilated as a positive element that contributed to the fulfilment of the desire for a child, without which this desire would not have been realised". For example, studies carried out in France with parents of children inseminated with anonymous semen show that, in cases of donation, paternity should be based on the relationship and not on physical resemblance (MANUEL apud CORRÊA, 2001, p. 184).

Some suggestions are made for overcoming the difficulties arising from treatments with reproductive technologies. Firstly, it is proposed that artificial procreation be accommodated to the current family and kinship model. Secondly, there is the idea of seeing artificial procreation not as a break with tradition, but as a possibility of realising a traditional and acceptable goal, which is to have children. In order to achieve this traditionally idealised dream, the users of these technologies must be able to put aside their reservations about the means with which they build their families and their kinship relationships, promoting a kind of covering of the techniques by tradition, emphasising the values of the family, parenthood and reproduction in order to circumvent the more controversial aspects of the process. In cases where the baby's intended parents resort to surrogacy, the establishment of an intense relationship between these parents and the surrogate during pregnancy, in an attempt to participate in the pregnancy, is very favourable. In the case of heterologous reproduction, the experience of raising the child, living with it on a day-to-day basis, is a strategy that can be positive (LUNA, 2002).

In my opinion, the most sensitive point of AR's effect on kinship lies in the "interference with the supposed biological truth" of the child, when a reality is created in which the social father and mother are different from the biological parents and even from the gestational mother (SALÉM, 1995), which is made worse by the concealment of the situation, which will invariably be part of both the life story of each of those involved and the process of building kinship ties. The concealment of facts does not transform or erase them and, as a way of overcoming probable tensions, all that remains is acceptance and living through the experience.

Another aspect of its relevance in the field of procreation through conceptual reproductive technologies is that it promotes the deconstruction of social notions , such as family and kinship, and also reinforces socially valued ideas, such as the categories of sex, gender and race, which are based on the differences in procedures between semen and egg donations.

2.3 **Reinforcing the notions of sex and gender**

Due to the differences between the two types of gamete donation (eggs and semen), as shown in the material presented in section 1.2 of this thesis, some scholars on the subject attribute different levels to the acts. Evidence of this is that in most countries, the law allows the donation of sperm and prohibits the donation of female reproductive cells. Furthermore, according to its collection, storage and shipping parameters, sperm is often compared to disposable products, which would make it easier to naturalise this type of donation (ALLEBRANDT, 2008).

According to Strathern (1995a), the issue implicit in the difference in treatment received by male and female gametes goes beyond the objectivity of the techniques. For the author, in addition to the distinction of the procreative role, the importance of the meanings attributed to the figures of father and mother for the construction of parenthood seems to be at stake, in which the female gamete would be related to hegemonic narratives about motherhood that affirm that "there is only one mother".

Konrad's (2005) reflections on RA in England make the same point: she believes that the distinction between egg donation and semen donation lies in the fact that the eggs have a shared biographical trajectory with the women who carry them, which is linked to reproduction and caring for offspring.

British scientist Erica Haimes carried out studies on human reproductive technologies and sex and gender issues. Her research began in the 1980s and aimed to understand the behaviour of British people in relation to these technologies, in terms of reproduction and the family, as well as to provide support for the state, with a view to building regulatory criteria for human fertilisation and embryology. The research data comes from two sources: the first refers to the detailed analyses of the English committee, the Wamock Report, which investigated the issue in question on national territory and compared the results with historical data from other governments. The second source of data was obtained through in-depth interviews with members of the Wamock Committee [15].

According to Haimes, "[...] the gender aspects of gamete donation are not immediately apparent, since semen and egg donation are often described as being essentially the same [...]" (HAIMES, 1997, p. 85). However, it was noted that alongside this position of equivalence there is a set of irregular assumptions about their differences. These assumptions are linked to ideas about the ways in which women and men are associated with reproduction and the family.

The analysis of the data obtained in the studies coordinated by Haimes suggests that, historically, semen donation has been associated with individualism, irregular behaviour and dubious sexual connotations, while egg donation has been related to altruism, the family, medicalisation and the absence of sexuality. These distinctions between the two types of donation work on many levels, but would be more pronounced in two aspects: the *donation procedures* and the *donors' motives.*

According to the research carried out, the motives behind gamete donors differ between the sexes. The intentions of male donors are seen as dubious, questionable and self-centred, possibly because they are associated with "deviant" sexuality: masturbation, adultery and illegitimacy, but also because of the "active" position that men have in the act. "[...] They may want to donate semen because they want to be fathers to many children, invading the families that their semen helps to create, which perhaps involves a high level of self-centredness, an illicit pleasure. [...]" (HAIMES, 1993, p. 91).

Unlike men, egg donors are seen as very altruistic, non-sexual, passive and family-orientated. They don't donate eggs, they lend themselves as subjects not only for the clinical procedures of egg collection, itself a more passive term than "donation", but they are also seen as victims of the medicalisation and exploitation of the medical clinic. Thus, the egg donor would be at risk of physical harm due to her direct participation in the practice of gamete extraction, serving to emphasise the view that her motives must be altruistic.

Symbolically, sperm and egg donation are also experienced differently among

[15] The Wamock Committee was also dealt with in section 2.3 of this project.

infertile couples. One study showed that 86% (eighty-six percent) of the women who were going to undergo heterologous insemination and 66% (sixty-six percent) of the partners receiving gametes were in favour of the possibility of recruiting the parties' sisters for egg donation, but only 9% (nine percent) of the women and 14% (fourteen percent) of the men expressed the same preference for siblings as semen donors (Yvon et al., 2004, p. 304). It's interesting to note the subjects' preference for egg donors, even though the procedure of extracting the material involves a highly invasive technique and poses risks for them, compared to semen donation which is free of health damage as it only involves masturbation.

These results can be analysed from various angles. Throughout the ages, women have occupied antagonistic positions: both as bearers of a negative nature and linked to the domestic, which is the domain of the sacred, which justifies the greater acceptance of egg donation compared to semen donation, since in this act the female sex is associated with both motherhood and illness, with sterility (HERTZ, 1980; ROHDEN, 2003). The paradox in which the female sex finds itself would be "resolved" through the logic of the "sanctification" of women, which in turn is linked to their asexualisation. Thus, motherhood and the mother-child relationship are valued and understood as natural facts.

The concept of natural motherhood was present both in the legal discourse defining the mother by childbirth, and in the idea of a female nature centred on reproduction and manifested in the maternal instinct, as constructed by 18th and 19th century medicine (ROHDEN, 2003).

From another perspective, as a mother, the woman would be a symbol of self-sacrifice, endowed with a peculiar nuance in the Brazilian case, where this position is doubly sacralised, according to two strands of values: the Mediterranean complex of honour and shame, which sacralises the "wife-mother" category, the focus of cooperation within the family, but mainly in maternal sexual virtue as a symbol of family honour and the moral solidarity of the group, showing herself to be selfless, self-sacrificing and protective (ARAGÃO, 1983). The second strand refers to the importance of Catholicism in shaping Brazilian values, placing the figure of the Virgin Mary as a maternal reference. In the perception that motherhood was natural, the existence of a father was necessary to establish sociability (HEILBORN, 1991; LUNA, 2002).

On the other hand, this opens up two conflicts related to male infertility. On the one hand, we realise that a man's ability to impregnate a woman confers a certain social *status* on him and is inextricably linked to the affirmation of his virility. On the other hand, the fact that the woman with whom this man has affective-sexual ties is fertilised by another man's sperm can lead to conflicts based on the idea of adultery.

In addition, gender differences point to social differences, which include experiences of fatherhood and motherhood. Although women and men today seek and even realise a certain parallelism in everyday life (work inside and outside the home, expenses, childcare, etc.), there is still a "mismatch between traditional cultural patterns and the rules of capitalism's postulation of equality" (HEILBORN, 1991, p. 35-33). (HEILBORN, 1991, p. 35-36), as is the case with women's double shift, for example, which means that women are more responsible for aspects of the home, which includes caring for offspring, as well as everything related to them (offspring): conception and contraception.

According to Scavone (2004, p. 7), "the construction of a new male identity, integrating sexual and reproductive life, means a constant confrontation with the dominant objective and subjective structures, and is therefore a slow process", while decisions about reproduction, as well as its consequences, are more the responsibility of women. It can also be seen that the recurrence of disbelief in the effective involvement of men in the experience of fatherhood, in a way, reinforces their distance from the consequences of reproduction.

When it comes to conception, even that resulting from reproductive technologies, men also seem to remain in a second-order position: fatherhood has always been dependent on motherhood. Pregnancy is thus constructed as an object belonging to the feminine and excluded from the masculine. It is important to emphasise that this difference in biological maternity as a differentiating factor between motherhood and fatherhood is based on a Western view of the phenomenon, and is therefore a social construction. The quote below makes this clear:

> [...] from a subjective point of view, motherhood is a relationship of intense affection, precisely because its biological process, from the beginning of gestation, is confined to women's bodies, establishing a close bond of belonging, which, in a way, excludes men. According to Barbieri (1990, p. 32): 'We, women and men, are essential for fertilisation, but only women's bodies have so far ensured [...] the survival of the fertilised body and therefore of the human species'. Perhaps this is one of the most important factors that differentiates motherhood from fatherhood [...] (SCAVONE, 2004, p. 5).

These differences between man/woman, paternity/maternity are identified in the legislative models of various countries, based on the permissions and prohibitions of techniques for conception via reproductive technologies. Generally speaking, the various pieces of legislation seen above are based on recognising that the legal bond of maternal filiation is established through childbirth, while paternity depends on the recognition of a social relationship in order to be established. This idea may explain the differences found in the treatment of egg and semen donations, which are based on cultural aspects (LUNA, 2002).

2.4 **Assisted reproduction: some questions about "race"**

As well as reproducing the social model of sex and gender, conceptive reproductive technologies also reinforce issues relating to "race", which is due to the fact that insemination with gamete donation involves the selection of a third individual in the reproduction process: the semen donor and/or the egg donor. The criteria used and the way in which the donor is chosen seem to reflect notions of "race", ethnicity and nationality. The following quote offers some thoughts on these categories:

> "Race" is a notion in which phenotypical characteristics such as skin colour, hair type, nose shape, lip thickness, among others, are used as parameters for classification. However, these characteristics only have meaning within a pre-existing ideology, an ideology that creates facts by relating them to each other. It is only because of and within this established relationship that these characteristics function as criteria and classification marks (GUIMARÃES, 1995). Thus, the marks matter precisely insofar as they represent differences in relation to other people, differences that translate, above all, into social inequalities (APPIAH, 1997). The notion of "race" points to the belief that bodies are privileged spaces for inscriptions and meanings (KOFES, 1996), although the word "race" should always be understood as designating any discussion of the term and the subject (COSTA, 2004, p. 236).

In a study carried out in the interior of São Paulo, researcher Suely Gomes da Costa analysed notions about "race" among doctors and patients waiting for an egg donor. The research also involved two São Paulo semen banks.

The research showed how the notion of "race" is linked to the idea of blood, which is now associated with or replaced by the idea of genes. The phenotypic characteristics categorised by the notion of "race" are understood by the doctors and patients interviewed as being transmitted by blood. This transmission through donated gametes is highly regulated by semen banks, but above all by the medical institution, which is both responsible for regulating the selection of gamete donors and for categorising donors according to its own criteria (COSTA, 2004).

Thus, despite the fact that there is a whole discussion inside and outside academia about racial classification in Brazil, medical institutions don't seem to be afflicted by this problem, and classify the donor candidates who go to the semen banks without any doubts, problems or questions. This is the case with the doctor in charge of one of the semen banks, who said: "I look at the donor and I can see straight away if he's black, or mulatto, or white". At both banks, according to the doctors interviewed, the majority of donors are "Caucasian" and the most sought-after semen is from "white" donors. Black" donors are few because there is little demand for their semen (COSTA,

2004, p. 235).

According to Costa, who interviewed the coordinators of the two semen banks, sperm from "black" donors is less in demand because "black" people have a lower socio-economic level and therefore don't have access to buying semen because of its high cost. The inverted commas in the words quoted above serve not only to indicate that they are part of the interviewed doctors' speech, but also to point to the issue of racial classification in the country.

According to the scholar, the categorisation of medical institutions in terms of colour and "race" is also informed by the relationship that *is* established between the doctor interviewing the donor candidate and the candidate; between the position of status/power of the doctor and that of the donor candidate, established by their age, education, profession etc. The same can be said for the choice of egg donor, which depends on the phenotypical classification of both the donor and the recipient, made by the doctor or medical team. Thus, the classification of colour and "race" in semen banks is already a filter carried out by medical institutions, which define *who* and what it is to be white, black, mulatto, light mulatto, dark mulatto; to have light or medium white skin, etc.

It can be seen in both semen banks that racial categories can be used as colour categories (mulatto), just as colour categories can be used as racial categories (white, black, yellow, brown). Categories of ethnic origin can be used as racial categories (Hispanic), just as one can be taken for the other (Italian for white). On an empirical level, this points to fusions and confusions regarding the notions of "race", colour and ethnicity (COSTA, 2004).

According to the interviews carried out in the research in question, it emerged that the patients who were going to undergo IVF with egg donation wanted donors who physically resembled them for various reasons:

1) Because children always look like their parents. Thus, the desire for children who look like the recipient appears as a prerogative of motherhood brought about by the use of reproductive technologies, since it is considered that if the child were not to look like the recipients, one would adopt one instead of resorting to assisted reproduction.

2) So that the child doesn't have any problems later on.

3) Because many couples keep the donation a secret and a child who doesn't look the same could reveal that secret.

However, despite the fact that these women initially related their desire for physical resemblance to the child to a fear of future conflicts, they later considered that if the donor was lighter than them, there wouldn't be a problem. According to one of them:

> I trust the hospital staff, that they'll find a good donor for me. But I wouldn't complain if the child came out blonde with blue eyes, which is so beautiful (COSTA, 2004, p. 247).

Even in cases where family and friends know about the donation, which leads to greater acceptance of the phenotypical differences between parents and children, this difference tends to whiten the child.

In the case of the other interviewees - who only told their mother, their best friend or didn't tell anyone - the issue of colour was also present when they justified their desire for a phenotypically similar donor, referring to the child's suffering when they realised they were different from their parents. However, concern was expressed about a child who was "darker" than the recipient or the recipient couple:

> We think about the child, when they start to understand things and then you have to explain to them why they're different, they can suffer. I've seen adoption cases where there are problems with colour. When the child starts to understand, they want to know why they're darker. They'll want to know why they're different, where they come from, the others will find it strange (COSTA, 2004, p. 247).

According to another patient: "People look at it differently, that's the way the world is. I have nothing against it. But there's racism, people stand in the adoption queue for ages and don't want to adopt a black child. If it's their turn and the child is black, they don't want to. (COSTA, 2004, p. 248).

In other words, it's other people who look at the child differently, it's other people who are considered prejudiced and racist. For the interviewees, this justifies their desire not to have a child with skin darker than their own, because they don't want the child to suffer this kind of prejudice. On the other hand, the justification given for other people not wanting darker-skinned children or not adopting black children is that they are racist and prejudiced. Thus, prejudice and racism always appear to be allocated to the Other. In this sense, it was considered that if the child at least looked like her husband, that was good enough. But, in any case, "not too dark". According to one of the interviewees:

> I'm light with green eyes and brown hair, and my husband is on the dark side sunburnt. So if the donor is too dark, the child won't look like me or my husband. It would be very different from me and him, and I wouldn't accept it. But if she's not very dark, then the child could look like the father, like the father, then there's no problem." (COSTA, 2004, p. 248).

The data collected in Costa's study shows that, although IVF with gamete donation is not used with the explicit purpose of affirming or denying characteristics considered to be racial/ethnic by the interviewees, it is very relevant and revealing that a child "lighter" than themselves can be accepted, while a "darker" child is rejected. It seems that, in a process of reflexive projection, a lighter child is seen as being able to contribute to "lightening" their own mother, their own family.

"In specific socio-cultural contexts, supposedly 'racial' characteristics can, of course, be highly predictive of social or cultural traits" (APPIAH apud COSTA, 2004, p. 249). In the Brazilian case, the effects of racial discrimination can be seen in the data relating to the black population's lower access to education, health and well-paid jobs, which contribute to "race" being a determining factor in social exclusion (FUNDAÇÃO... apud COSTA, 2004, p. 249). In the *ranking* of quality of life measured by the Human Development Index (HDI), black Brazilians are in 101st place, while white Brazilians are in 46th place (FOLHA... apud COSTA, 2004, p. 249-250). Oliveira (apud COSTA, 2004, p. 250) cites the higher perinatal, neonatal and infant mortality among the black population and the drastically increasing numbers of young black people who have been victims of violent deaths, especially in metropolitan regions. Araújo (apud COSTA, 2004, p. 250) refers to the problems relating to black people's self-esteem generated by an ideology of whitening.

The interviewees' attribution of racial prejudice to others (society, neighbours, school) shows how taboo this subject is. In this sense, data from a survey carried out in the 1990s shows that while 89 per cent (eighty-nine per cent) of those interviewed thought that Brazilians are racist, only 10 per cent (ten per cent) said that they themselves were racist (MELO; TURRA; VENTURI apud COSTA, 2004, p. 250).

Assisted reproduction allows some elements of the model considered to be natural reproduction, such as having sex, transmitting genes and giving birth, to be preserved (STRATHERN apud COSTA, 2004, p. 251). Thus, if in assisted reproduction with gamete donation there is no sexual intercourse or transmission of genetic characters, the phenotypic similarity acts as a symbolic substitute for the transmission of genes (by one or both of the couple's components), which can mask/hide/make irrelevant the fact that this transmission has not occurred. Donation also allows pregnancy and childbirth to be preserved. On the other hand, adopting a child is seen as a second option because it doesn't allow any of these elements to be preserved.

For Costa, if we agree with the idea that similarity is in the eye of the beholder, we have to consider that the ideal donor is the one who makes it possible for the recipient to establish desirable similarities, selected from the variety of characteristics present in the recipients themselves and their relatives. But what ends up prevailing in this selection are the classifications made by medical institutions, with the aim of regulating that gamete donations and receptions are made between those considered similar.

In the next chapter we will look at the theory of gift. Since this research was analysed using this theoretical framework, which served as a guide to better understanding the phenomenon of the reasons that move a man to donate semen, we will then present some considerations about the studies systematised by Mareei Mauss, the reflections made by intellectuals in the field, and end with contemporary analyses of the modern gift.

CHAPTER 3

THE GIFT

> [...] there is a series of rights and duties to consume and reciprocate, corresponding to rights and duties to give and receive. However, this close mix of symmetrical and contrary rights and duties no longer seems contradictory if we consider that, first and foremost, there is a mix of spiritual bonds between things, which are to a certain extent soul, and individuals and groups, which treat each other to a certain extent as things. And all these institutions express only one fact, one social regime, one defined mentality: that everything, food, women, children, goods, talismans, land, labour, services, priestly offices and posts are a matter of transmission and retribution. Everything goes back and forth as if there were a constant exchange of spiritual matter comprising things and men, between clans and individuals, divided between categories, sexes and generations (MAUSS, 1974, p. 59).

Mareei Mauss, a French sociologist and anthropologist, presented unprecedented and relevant reflections on the gift in his famous work *Essair sur le don,* translated as *Essay on the Gift,* which systematised a theory on the phenomenon. The work was first published in 1924 and is reproduced in a collection entitled *Sociologia e antropologia*, published in Brazil in 1974. Academics unanimously consider the *Essay to* be a masterpiece, as well as Mauss' main work. This *essay,* of immense fruitfulness for the formulation of theories on the nature of social life, was responsible for countless debates in the social sciences, by demonstrating the multiplicity of aspects - political, social, economic, religious, etc. - that are closely linked to gift systems. Gift here is not to be confused with the common sense translation of the term. In Brazil, for example, it is mainly identified with the Catholic ideas of charity and blessing, reducing the gift to a religious phenomenon. Although charity and blessing correspond to a certain type of gift, for the author, the term has a broader meaning: an organisational logic of the social that has a universalising character, in which the gift appears as a moral rule that is imposed on the community.

The *Essay on the Gift* is part of a series of studies that Mauss began on archaic forms of contract and, in particular, on the *potlatch*[16] . In addition, the author draws on data from students and collaborators (ethnologists, anthropologists and missionaries),

[16] In some Native American tribes of the Pacific Northwest region of the United States and Canada, *potlatch is* a ritual practice in which men use gifts as a way of indicating their *status* in relation to other men. It is a form of bravado intended to demonstrate how wealthy and generous a given man is, at the expense of those receiving the gifts. The recipients, for their part, feel obliged to act in the same way at some point in the future, so that they can move on to a higher position (JOHNSON, 1997, p. 179-180).

collected in studies of so-called "traditional", non-capitalist societies, mainly in Melanesia and the American north-west; he also establishes a comparison with "some features of Indo-European rights": Roman, classical Hindu and Germanic law. His attention turns to a set of apparently free and gratuitous benefits, but which are, as he shows, obligatory and interested.

In the *Essay,* Mauss sought to demonstrate that the phenomena of the state and the market are not universal, since no evidence was found of their presence in "traditional" societies, but only in more complex societies, such as modern ones. However, it was found that in all existing societies, regardless of whether they are traditional or modern, there is a constant presence of a system of interpersonal reciprocities. This system appears as a total social phenomenon, cutting across the whole of social life, to the extent that everything that participates in human life, be it goods or gestures, is relevant to the production of society.

The leitmotif of the work is the notion of "alliance". Mauss argues that the gift produces *an* alliance, both *matrimonial* alliances (unions between people) and *political* alliances (exchanges between chiefs or between different social strata; what emerges when exchanges are unsuccessful, resulting in war; the exchange of violence; or the imbalance between what is exchanged, etc.), *religious* (such as sacrifices, understood as a way of relating to the gods), as well as *economic* alliances, *legal* alliances, *diplomatic* alliances (including personal relationships of hospitality), and *aesthetic* alliances (present in the making of objects, the way they are offered, etc.).

Mauss proposes a reflection on the phenomenon from a broad perspective. For him, exchange includes not only gifts but also visits, feasts, communions, alms, inheritances, women and a multitude of "instalments" - instalments that can be "total" (referring to everything that is exchanged) or "agonistic" (a type of exchange that involves a struggle).

The main thesis of the *Essay* refers to an understanding of the constitution of social life by a constant give and take, based on a tension between obligation and spontaneity in the universe of exchanges. The study shows how, universally, giving and giving back are obligations, but organised in a particular way in each situation and group. Hence the importance of understanding how exchanges are conceived and practised in different times and places, as well as the different forms they take, ranging from personal retribution to the redistribution of taxes. According to the author:

> Of all these very complex themes and this multiplicity of social things in motion, we want to consider a single, profound, but isolated feature: the voluntary character, so to speak, apparently free and gratuitous, and yet

imposed and interested, of these services (MAUSS, 1974, p. 41).

Mauss points to the fact that some exchanges are the prerogatives of leaders: receiving tribute, for example. These prerogatives are socially constructed and, as such, vary from society to society, such as: via privileges, via obligations, etc. To this, the author associated the fact that leadership often emanates values that extend to societies as a whole, becoming generalised. However, the generative or sociability-creating aspect of the gift is not limited to politics. In the epigraph to his work, he expresses a dialectic inherent to the gift: when receiving a visitor, the subject is making himself a host, but at the same time, theoretically and conceptually, he is creating the possibility of becoming a guest of the person who is currently his guest. The logic of the gift dialectic points to the following "equation": the same exchange that makes a subject a host also makes them a potential guest. This is because "giving and receiving" implies not only a material exchange, but also a spiritual exchange, a communication between souls, whose dimension is much broader than the utilitarian vision of the gift.

It is in this ontological sense of gift theory that every exchange presupposes some kind of alienability, because when you give, you always give something of yourself; when you accept, the recipient accepts something from the giver. And although the gift produces inequalities, when something is given from one person to another and the other reciprocates, albeit momentarily, they cease to be independent individuals. At that moment, the gift has brought the parties closer together, making them similar and interconnected.

In addition, the circulation of material-immaterial goods can imply greater or lesser alienability in terms of what is exchanged, in other words, the relationship between greater and lesser alienability and the creation of value is not something simple and straightforward, but rather varies over time and space. Mauss called the described scheme of voluntary, but strictly obligatory, benefits and rewards *a system of total benefits,* which refers to voluntary benefits and rewards.

Mareei Mauss formulated a key idea from which the phenomenon of the circulation of gifts and counter-gifts, encompassing various domains of collective life, came to be analysed based on the concept of the *total social fact.* The notion of the *total social fact* included a concern to examine the relationships between the physiological, psychological and social aspects of the human being in an integrated way. The phenomenon is evident in the most different civilisations, which show us that exchange allows communication between men, inter-subjectivity, sociability, according to rules that establish it. These rules manifest themselves simultaneously in morality, literature, law, religion, economics, politics, the organisation of kinship and the aesthetics of different societies, among others. You can isolate the economic aspect of an exchange, but it always involves, at the same time, a religious aspect, a political aspect or even an aesthetic aspect, as described above.

> The notion of a total social fact refers to a certain type of ceremonial exchange - material and symbolic - which simultaneously activates various levels (religious, economic, legal and moral, aesthetic, morphological) of a society. Thus, from an analytical point of view, total social facts would be more than themes or elements of institutions; more than complex institutions or even systems of religious, legal, economic or other institutions. Total social facts would represent the social system itself in operation (MAUSS, 1974, p. 145).

To formulate the concept of the *total social fact,* Mauss took as his basis the earlier sociological concept of the *social fact,* presented by Émile Durkheim, considered one of the founders of sociology along with Karl Marx and Max Weber. The sociologist pointed to the peculiarity of society as an object of scientific study, as a "thing", excluding a purely psychological approach to facts. Durkheim proposed a positivist, scientific analysis of facts, as was the case with the theme of "suicide" developed in his work *Rules of the Sociological Method* (1895). Mauss introduced the symbolic aspect to Durkheim's concept, going beyond the limits of positivism. In other words, in *total social facts* - such as exchange in the tribes of the American north-west - religious, legal, moral and economic institutions are expressed, as well as the aesthetic and morphological aspects of the phenomenon. In short, all of social life is mixed up and present there.

Following Mauss, the act of giving would not be a disinterested act, in other words, there would be no such thing as a gift without the expectation of retribution, nor would it be limited to the practice of "chiefs", but would extend to the community. This means that in addition to the mixture of souls and things, the sociability in the act of exchange, and the coercive character embedded in altruism, since you don't have the right to refuse a gift, it would be made up of a triple obligation: to give, to receive and to reciprocate. In this mixture of people and things, the consideration would be equivalent to a new instalment that would require a new retribution. "To refrain from giving, like refraining from receiving, is to lose one's dignity - like refraining from giving back." (MAUSS, 1974, p. 111).

In order to find an explanation for the dynamics of the gift, and making reference to the testimony of a Maori informant extracted from the notes of the ethnographer Robert Hertz, Mareei Mauss attributes to the notion of hau a justification for the circulation of gifts. The author explains this notion as follows:

> I'm going to tell you about the *hau...* The *hau* is not the wind that blows. Not at all. Suppose you have a certain item [taonga], and you give it to me: you give it to me without a fixed price. We don't do business with that. Now, I give that item to a third person who, after a while, decides to give something in payment [utu], giving me something [taonga]. Now, this *taonga* that he gives me is the spirit [hau] of *taonga* that I received from you and that I gave to him. The *taonga* I received for those *taonga* [from the lord] I have to give back to him. It wouldn't be fair [tika] of me to keep these *taonga* for myself, whether they are desirable [rawe] or unpleasant [kino]. I must give them to you, because they are a *hau* of *taonga* that you had given me. If I were to keep this second *taonga* for myself, it could bring me serious harm, even death. Such is the *hau* of personal property, the *hau of taonga,* the *hau* of the forest. *Kati ena* [enough on the subject] (MAUSS, 1974, p. 53).

The exchange of gifts takes place because "giving and receiving" implies not only a material exchange, but also a spiritual exchange, a communication between souls, which is part of the notion of *hau.* The dimension of this type of immaterial exchange would be much broader than the utilitarian vision of the gift present in modern societies, according to the author. It is mainly at this point that Mauss' sociology reveals itself to be a sociology of the symbol. On the other hand, it was also at this point that his work raised the most questions.

3.1 **Some considerations on Maussian thought**

At the time of its publication, the *Essay on the Gift* was well accepted by academics. However, some time later, because Mauss accepted the native explanation of the spiritual bond between things and people, some criticisms emerged. Anthropologist Raymond Firth criticised Mauss' *essay* in his work *Primitive Economics of the New Zealand Maori* (1929). The main aspect addressed concerned the concept of *hau* which, according to Firth, did not refer to the spirit of the giver, but to the spirit of the thing, suggesting that Mauss had allowed himself to be influenced by the indigenous people.

Anthropologist Claude Lévi-Strauss (1974), in his introduction to the work of Mareei Mauss, emphasises the importance and contribution of the *Essay* to anthropology and science. However, while paying tribute to the originality and relevance of Mauss' anthropological project, Lévi-Strauss harshly criticises the explanation proposed in the book.

An essay on the obligatory nature of reciprocity, from which it becomes clear that there is a disagreement as to the nature of the anthropological endeavour and the *status* to be attributed to "native explanations".

Lévi-Strauss points to the introduction of the idea of the *total social fact as* the greatest theoretical contribution of the *Essay.* However, the place attributed to the social should be examined, according to the author. For him, the social, according to Mauss, would be reality. But in fact, the social could only be real if it met a double condition: firstly, it had to be integrated into a system, which spoke of the countless aspects into which social life can be broken down by scholars. Secondly, it had to be embodied in an individual experience. According to Lévi-Strauss, the *total social fact* would be "three-dimensional", presenting sociological, historical and physiopsychological aspects, thus requiring a flesh and blood individual in which to materialise. Only through the study of concrete individual experiences would the social fact be apprehensible.

Mauss would have resorted to the native Maori theory of the *hau* to justify his reflections on exchange because of the real impossibility of attributing it to a physical property inherent in the objects exchanged. It was at this point that Lévi-Strauss placed his critical view of Mauss' work, since "the *hau* is not the ultimate reason for exchange: it is the conscious way in which the men of a particular society, where the problem was of particular importance, apprehended an unconscious necessity whose reason lies elsewhere." (LÉVI-STRAUSS, 1974, p. 25-26).

In this sense, it would be up to the anthropologist to go beyond the explanations contained in the discourse of the natives, since what "those concerned (...) believe they think or do is always far removed from what they actually think or do". (Idem, p. 26). Following his reflections, the ethnographic research project then aims to reach an "underlying reality", unconscious in the native mind and accessible preferably through the examination of institutions and language - the unconscious mental structures, more suitable access routes for the search of that underlying reality than its "conscious elaborations". After all, there is much more to exchange than the things exchanged, which carry with them processes of group formation and profit translated into non-economic currencies, such as power, prestige and affection.

Pierre Bourdieu, in *Ésquisse dune theorie de la pratique*[17] (1972), proposes the resolution of the opposition between Mauss and Lévi-Strauss by integrating someone's perception of their practice with the logic that underlies it. Bourdieu realises that the essence of the opposition lies in the fact that Mauss discusses the present as it was

[17] The references of this work translated into Portuguese are: BOURDIEU, Pierre. *Outline of a theory of practice.* Oeiras: Celta, p. 265

experienced, while Lévi-Strauss examines it outside of its everyday insertion. The present, for those who experience it, is spontaneous and disinterested. However, for those who observe it from the outside, it seems forced and motivated by interest.

Bourdieu notes that there was nothing wrong with the two observations, just different points of view and different observation times. The author introduces the idea of the *temporal dimension,* which is the time elapsed between the gift and the counter-gift, ignored by objectivism, as the element that makes possible the coexistence of two opposing truths - disinterest and calculation - between the native and external views of the gift system.

By examining the debate between Lévi-Strauss and Mauss, Pierre Bourdieu takes a decisive step towards developing the central elements of his sociology: the perception of social structures which, when incorporated by agents, come to guide their actions.

Bourdieu's concept of *habitus*, which designates a system of structured structures predisposed to function as structuring structures, in other words, a kind of social introjected and recreated by each individual's mental apparatus, which produces an intersection between the coercion of the social that structures and is structured by each human being, served as a reference in the question of the dynamics of giving. Bourdieu comes close to Mauss' notion of a set of collective expectations and proposes that the system could be understood as a "collective self-deception", since the generosity that drives the gift is anchored in the donor's assumption that their act will be understood as generous and rewarding.

It's important to note that the *Essay* allows Mauss to touch the "concrete", to highlight the central mechanism of solidarity which is reciprocity, to criticise the utilitarianism of economic theories and to extract a heuristic principle which consists of studying facts as "total social facts". For him, this is a way of "touching one of the human rocks on which our societies are built". Mauss' merit was to demonstrate that the life of the 'primitive' is more complex, more active and more dynamic than we believe. That's why it's necessary not to represent it as "static". Furthermore, economic life seems to be deeply linked to morality and religiosity. According to Mauss, everything is in everything.

The *Essay on the Gift is* so important and central to Mauss' work that it was a meeting point between his scientific and political concerns. Furthermore , according to Allain Caillé, Mauss' theory "provides the guidelines not only for one sociological paradigm among others, but for the only properly sociological paradigm that can be conceived and defended." (CAILLÉ, 1998, p. 11). For him, by demonstrating that the social has its own rules that cannot be reduced to utilitarian ones, Mauss would have broken with the defensive and ambiguous stance that sociology has traditionally taken towards the idea of *homo economicus.* As sociology, Mauss' work would also go beyond the limits of Durkheimian dualist representations to become a decisive theoretical resource for criticising the presence of utilitarian theses within the social sciences and for motivating a deeper discussion about the political and moral foundations of democracy.

Unlike his uncle Durkheim, who would have stuck to the scientific idea of objectifying social reality, Mauss realised that society is primarily instituted by a symbolic dimension, and that there is a close link between symbolism and the obligation to give, receive and reciprocate in all societies. On the other hand, one of his main merits would have been to overcome the dichotomies of Durkheim's theory (between the sacred and the profane, between the individual and society, between the normal and the pathological), to propose the hypothesis that society is a total phenomenon, at the same time as it is delineated by individual differences and their idiosyncrasies. At this point, Mauss introduces the idea of paradox, i.e. human motivations are necessarily paradoxical.

By emphasising the idea of a totality that is not merely an objectivist representation, but a symbolic one, dualistic and separatist dogmas are shattered. Thus, society comes to be understood as a whole made up of circulating meanings (gestures, laughter, words, gifts, sacrifices, etc.); the sociological analysis of social reality must not only take into account the multiple signs/symbols that articulate the actors and social institutions in one and the same network, but critical analysis must also be open to a complex understanding of experience. This perspective of a totality that is ambivalent implies that the creation of the social bond occurs within social practices, "from their environment, horizontally, as a function of the set of interrelationships that link individuals and transform them into properly social actors." (CAILLÉ, 2000, p. 19). For Mauss, what circulates influences how actors are formed and how their places in society are defined.

According to Jacques Godbout, who continues to theorise about the gift, Maussian thought has its own rules. It is a genuine social system, with specificities that differentiate it from other systems existing in society. In this sense, "it is important to observe, as a priority in everyday life, not the actors and structures, but what circulates between the actors in favour of the social bond: the material and symbolic goods that society has at its disposal to reproduce itself through the actors that make it up."

(GODBOUT, 1999, p. 23).

According to the author, the gift is present everywhere and doesn't just concern isolated and discontinuous moments in reality. What circulates has many names: it's called money, cars, furniture, real estate, clothes, but also smiles, kindness, words, hospitality, gifts, free services, as well as donations of human material that have been widely used, such as blood, organs for transplantation and reproductive cells, considered by today's scholars to be modern gifts.

3.2 **Modern gift**

> The modern person frees himself from attachments to people by replacing them, as far as possible, with attachments to things, certainly saying that this is much less imposing, since it's easier to separate from a cat or a dog than from a child [...].
>
> The modern person, pseudo-emancipated from the duty of reciprocity, collapses under the weight of the accumulation of what he receives without giving back, he becomes sick, and his sensitivity makes him unable to bear human relationships. A vulnerable being who has lost his immune defence system against negative relationships, running away from the give-receive-return cycle for fear of being deceived, "asepticising" the cycle into one-sided, objective, precise, calculable, mechanical, predetermined, accountable, explicit, objectified, cold relationships.... whereas, as we have seen, to give back is to give, to give is to receive and to give back, to receive is to give; to give, to receive, to give back is to always be placing the indeterminacy of the world and the risk of existence, it is to always be making society, all of society, exist (GODBOUT, 1999, p. 252-253).

Jacques Godbout has made an important contribution to reflections on the gift in current times, continuing, according to his own interpretation, Mareei Mauss' endeavour at the point where it was interrupted: at the gates of modernity. He argues that the characteristics of modernity or post-modernity - a term used by the author, as well as by various intellectuals, to refer to the present moment, in terms of changes relating to the emergence of the state, the weakening of religion and community life, and the strengthening of science and individualism, the spread of technology and its impact on life in society, among others - would be incongruous with the gift and the humanitarianism that characterises it, a priori. However, the author proposes that the gift, as a type of social bond, should be detached from the economic logic to which it is usually linked and started to be thought of as a relationship, because this is where we would find the obstacle to linking the notion of the gift to the exchanges that take place in so-called Western societies, to what the author calls "selfish moralism". The quote below illustrates this:

> If modernity refuses to believe in the existence of the gift, it is because it represents it as the inverted image of selfish material interest. In its eyes, the "true" gift could only be free. And since gratuitousness is impossible *("There is no such*

> *thing as a free lunch*", and no one will ever shave for free), the gift, the true gift, is equally impossible. Hence, on the other hand, the insistence of those who are effectively dedicated to claiming that they, too, benefit from the gift. On the one hand, [...] this allows them to submit to the selfish moralism of the time. However, in essence, by denying the gratuitousness of their motivations, they attest to the reality of their gift. In fact, as Mary Douglas (1989) shows, the free gift doesn't really exist - or else in a way that is asymptotic to sociality. For the gift serves, first and foremost, to establish relationships. And a relationship with no hope of return (on the part of the giver or someone else who replaces them), a one-way relationship, gratuitous in this sense and for no reason, would not be a relationship. Beyond or below the abstract moments of egoism and altruism, the antithesis fixed between a moment considered real of calculated material interest and a moment considered ideal but inaccessible of radical disinterest, we need to think of the gift not as a series of unilateral and discontinuous acts, but as a relationship. [...] (GODBOUT, 1999, p. 15-16).

According to the researcher, the "dissonance" between the gift and modernity would contribute to maintaining the association of the phenomenon with "primitive" societies and, consequently, as a target of greater interest for anthropology, compared to sociology. On the contrary, he proposes the hypothesis that "the gift does not only concern primitive societies, but also contemporary society, albeit in a modified way that still needs to be analysed. (GODBOUT, 1999, p. 28). For him, the desire to give is just as important for understanding today's man as the desire to receive, because:

> [that compassion and generosity are as essential as taking, appropriating or conserving, as envy or selfishness. Or that "the seduction of the gift" has as much or more power than the seduction of gain, and that it is therefore as essential to elucidate its rules as it is to know the laws of the market or of bureaucracy in order to understand modern society [...] (GODBOUT, 1999, p. 28).

The author argues that in modern societies, as well as in ancient or traditional ones, there is a form of circulation of goods that differs intrinsically from the form analysed by economists. Through the gift, goods circulate at the service of bonds. The gift would act as the gift of a good or service with no guarantee of return, with a view to creating, nurturing or recreating social bonds between people. In a gift system, the pleasure of giving back has to be at stake, in other words, the value is in the relationship. In a market system, goods are worth between themselves and the relationship doesn't need to exist. Thus, faced with the risks inherent in any gift, money and recourse to a mercantilist logic are the antidotes, at the same time as they are counter-donations and poisons par excellence.

> [...] A gift is neither good nor bad in itself, nor is it always desirable. It all depends on the context of the relationship that gives it meaning. The market may be preferable. For example, you have no interest in accepting a gift from a person from whom you want to remain independent. The market is a unique social invention, and so is the state. The gift, since it is based more on trust

> than the market, is riskier, more dangerous and affects the person more deeply when the rules are not respected, when they allow themselves to be deceived [...] (GODBOUT, 1999, p. 238).

According to Godbout's analyses, in modern Western societies there are three main spheres where gifts circulate, based on different principles. These are: the *market, the state* and *the domestic sphere.* The principle that defines the market sphere is the possibility *and* ease of leaving the social relationship *(e.i'//)* in which an agent is not satisfied. The political sphere is, above all, governed by discussion and debate *(yoice)* . And it is "loyalty" that constitutes the basic principle of the domestic sphere, considered the natural place of the gift (GODBOUT, 1999, p. 33).

The commodity does not collude with the gift. In this sphere, agents make contact for the sole purpose of maximising their material interests. On the other hand, the ideology of the market favours breaking off the relationship when the good purchased does not satisfy. This is the model to which most consumers adapt.

In the case of the state sphere, the question is reversed. The development of the welfare state has been viewed favourably by many for reducing social injustices and restoring dignity to individuals, as opposed to previous redistribution systems based on charity. Nowadays, a significant proportion of the things and services that previously used the circuits of charity networks or personal ties between close people are accessible through the state and its distribution apparatus.

Many scholars agree that the state sphere could replace the gift in modern society, as the traditional forms of the gift are becoming more and more residual. Mareei Mauss believes that in Western society, the gift takes the form, above all, of redistribution by the state, that social security is in some way an extension of the primitive gift, and that the other manifestations of the gift, absent from this context, will end up being replaced in such a way that the traditional gift will be imbricated in one way or another in the action of the state. The payment of taxes would be an example of this.

Godbout emphasises the importance of the mixed forms of circulation (traditional gift and state "gift") resulting from state distribution for social life, but disagrees that the state sphere belongs to the universe of the gift. For him, this sphere is simply based on different principles, and in some situations it can even have negative effects on the gift. The author exemplifies his analysis with a current form of gift distribution: blood donation.

Unlike organ donation, blood donation is partly commercialised in many societies. The quote below illustrates this:

> [...] Here in Brazil, a company collects blood in order to treat haemophiliacs for free. At least that's what it advertises. And that's how it does it... in part. Because the amount of blood collected is so large that a considerable proportion - what's left over - is sold for other purposes. The system would collapse if the donors knew this (GODBOUT, 1999, p. 68).

Richard Titmuss (1972) researched the "modern gift" of blood donation. His analyses of the phenomenon were based on the relationship between strangers, which is generally mediated by the state in cooperation with the Red Cross. This type of donation calls into question the relationship generally established between gift and social ties, and has its own peculiar characteristics:

a. Firstly, anonymity favours the donor-recipient relationship, as it hides religious, political and ethnic issues, among others, which could be conflictive between the parties, or even hinder them, thus de-characterising the community-type relationship.

b. Secondly, blood donation is the responsibility of a system of paid intermediaries belonging to the state apparatus, and the blood is made available to the recipient thanks to this organisation, thus resembling all the other products received by a patient, occupying a certain place in the treatment, as is the case with serum and prescribed medication, for example. Thus, after the act of donation, blood becomes a product like all the others when it passes through the first recipient: the Red Cross.

c. Thirdly, the gift-poison is eminently present in the gesture of blood donation, because it is intrinsically always fraught with danger. In the past, hepatitis B was commonly transmitted through blood transfusions. Nowadays, the possibility of being infected with the AIDS virus is the most worrying aspect of the procedure.

In the United States, for example, self-donation is growing steadily, meaning that many people already collect blood and leave it on *standby* in specific banks for possible personal use in the future.

According to Godbout, based on the Maussian view, and due to the characteristics mentioned above, blood donation could not be qualified as a gift because there is no return on the part of the recipient. In this sense, the type of relationship that involves the blood donor and the recipient would be at odds with the "give-receive-return" circuit of the gift system formulated by Mauss.

Taking Sahlins (1976) and Hyde (1983) as a basis, the gift is characterised by the voluntary and free gesture, which is not always the case with blood donation, reinforcing its disqualification from the notion of gift.

In contrast, Titmuss concluded that this modern gift is a system based on giving and is therefore superior to the market, which Godbout proposes relativising for today. For Titmuss, this system is fundamentally different from the ancient gift, because it is a voluntary gift, with no obligation to return, and to a stranger. The scholar adds that these traits are characteristic of what circulates in the public sphere, and that the public system, unlike the market, would have the property of spreading the spirit of the gift in society, since government solidarity and the gift amplify and feed off each other (TITMUSS, 1972).

For Titmuss, the more society improves its standard of living, the more it will move from selling blood to donating it, as the dominant way of circulating the material. Whilst it is claimed that donation is an archaic form and that the market is the future for blood, the author inverts the usual reasoning because, for him, it is important to donate to strangers. "When the gift comes to include strangers, it brings about a change in values that reinforces the altruistic dimension of the gift relationship." (TITMUSS, 1972, p. 226). This possibility of donating to strangers is a characteristic of the modern gift and would be stimulated by the state, by the public responsibility assumed in the case of blood donation, which "allows ordinary people to consider the gesture of donation a moral value, even if it is outside their family structures and interpersonal relationships." (TITMUSS, 1972, p. 226).

Godbout says that Titmuss' theory is partly contradicted by what happens in industrialised countries, where the role of the state is the most important and blood tends to be sold rather than donated. In this sense, it is necessary to develop research that favours a better understanding of this issue.

The next chapter will present another approach to gamete donation, closer to the theme chosen in this study, which refers to heterologous assisted reproduction as a network of gifts. I propose that in it all the characters - conceptive technologies, professionals, users, semen donor, egg donor, surrogate mother and the resulting baby - build a system of gifts, which works in favour of one main gift: life.

CHAPTER 4

CONCEPTIVE REPRODUCTIVE TECHNOLOGIES: A NETWORK OF GIFTS?

The progress of modern Western medicine has been characterised by the continuous technological evolution of diagnostic and therapeutic methods aimed at achieving man's physical and mental well-being, or his "perfect health", by the control and discipline of human behaviour, by the logic of consuming medical acts and medicines, by the incessant search for monetary profits involving the pharmaceutical industry, health plans, insurance companies, clinics, hospitals, etc. This phenomenon has been called "social medicalisation", which is discussed in the second chapter of this thesis. In summary, the process of social medicalisation can be seen as the progressive expansion of biomedicine's field of intervention by redefining human experiences and behaviours as if they were medical problems (TESSER, 2006).

Taking another focus of analysis as a basis, which is very widespread among the anti-utilitarian movementM.*A.U.S.S*[18] ., two major currents of thought stand out, through which medical practices have also been scrutinised. These, apparently contradictory, are based on the oppositions between individualism and holism in the explanation of social facts and actions. One and the other rests on a visceral utilitarianism, according to which any and all social action is based on a web of interests, in other words, the links that are established in society and in people's daily lives are exhausted in an impersonal relationship of "supply and demand", regulated by money, in an exchange of equivalents (NUNES, 2004). According to Martins (2003), this is precisely the cause of the legitimacy crisis that medicine is going through.

In *Against the Dehumanisation of Medicine: A Sociological Critique of Modern Medical Practices*, sociologist Paulo Henrique Martins proposes a different view of the medical profession, based on the theory of the gift. Prioritising the social bond, the author demonstrates that the doctor-patient relationship is a social relationship, where other dimensions come into play, or *into* play, in which payment in money is just one of them (NUNES, 2004): "(...) Before being a set of techniques, medicine appears as a game of collective beliefs and rituals, created by each society to resolve the dilemma fundamental to human existence: that of life/death." (MARTINS, 2003, p.78).

[18] M.A.U.S.S. - Mouvement anti-utilitariste dans les Sciences socials. The material produced by the group is available at: http://www.revuedumauss.com. On 30/12/2009, at 19:28 pm.

According to the author, the introduction of alternative medicine at the end of the last century was a reaction to the harmful effects of the scientific and commercial utilitarianism of "traditional" medical practice, which neutralised the social nature of the profession. In this sense, alternative medicine is founded on a common root, the centrepiece of which is the paradigm of the gift.

> (...) alternative disciplines constitute a medical field of a different kind that finds its cement not in the control exercised by disciplinary organisation (faculties, laboratories, technicians, economic corporations, professional associations, etc.), but by valuing a medical education that is based on the experience lived spontaneously, freely, obliged and also interested in by the future therapist (MARTINS, 2003, p. 312).

In fact, "alternative" medicine has been understood as a phenomenon stemming from the counterculture movement of the 1960s, the meaning of which would be the reaction against the dehumanisation, commercialisation and mechanisation of "traditional" medicine. (RUSSO, 1993; MAGNANI, 2000). In my opinion, both types of medicine circulate between commerce and the gift, although each one shows closer links to one of the two phenomena. This means that neither "alternative" medicine is pure gift, nor "traditional" medicine is absolutely commercial. In some respects, "alternative" medicine has links to utilitarianism and, in turn, "traditional" medicine would establish links with the logic of generosity, since the latter is exercised in favour of human health and life, while in natural medicine - another name for "alternative" medicine -, significant amounts are also charged for consultations, treatments and products (essential oils, diffusers, handmade candles, CDs, DVDs, flower essences, aromatic pillows, crystals, relaxing slippers, clothing and a whole range of items for balancing the body, mind and spirit).

The topic in question, of alternative practices within Western medicine, is extremely relevant. However, I don't intend to delve deeper into discussions on the subject, since the aim of the research proposed here is to investigate the practice of donating male gametes in the context of assisted reproduction, based on the theory of the gift.

The bibliographical survey carried out for this study showed that research into AR tends to relate the field to the logic of the market. This chapter aims to discuss the two points of the phenomenon: commerce and the gift in the field of conceptual technologies.

4.1 Assisted reproduction: gift or trade?

Assisted reproduction is part of a field crossed by different forces, antagonistic in some respects. On the one hand, the practice is driven by altruism: realising the desire for a child of someone unable to conceive naturally. On the other hand, it is part of a context characterised by the power of specialists and industry, by profit and by services aimed at the more privileged social classes.

Various authors who have carried out research on the subject have concluded that reproductive technologies have some kind of link to the market, albeit in a veiled way. The context in which the practice takes place would end up producing a system of commercialisation of what is advertised as free, as well as a distinction in treatment between patients, whose financial *status* would be equally differentiated.

Based on a survey of doctors and patients from public and private clinics offering assisted reproduction services, anthropologist Rosely Gomes Costa (2006) found notable differences between the two types of healthcare area. The researcher exposes the commercial and non-ethical aspects that seem to surround the donation of reproductive cells, based on the differences identified with regard to the treatment offered to female patients in the public and private sectors.

Costa explains that while in the public health system immediate authorisation was given to keep in touch with the patients in order to get them to take part as interviewees, and a list of their names and telephone numbers was even provided, in the private health system the opposite was the case; contact with the patients was prevented. The doctors at these private clinics themselves refused to take part in the research, on the grounds that it would be embarrassing for the patient to talk about it, or because they felt that they would be forced to take part in the research, even if they didn't want to. However, in the past, some of these doctors had carried out their own master's and doctoral research with patients from the public health system, where, rather than interviews, body examinations were carried out, some of them quite invasive.

For the researcher, what seems to be being protected by private doctors is not the well-being of patients, but the satisfaction of their clients. The following quote illustrates the point:

> [...] The right to privacy and not to be embarrassed appears to be a good to be acquired, and the fear of doctors in private clinics of embarrassing their patients seems to be related more to the fear of losing clients than to a concern for the patient. In other words, the aim is to protect the private client, not the public patient (COSTA, 2006, p. 1).

This difference in treatment between the two types of patients can be seen in any medical speciality, and is not specific to the area of assisted reproduction, but it is clearly perceived in this area, due to the embarrassment attributed or felt in relation to the subject. For the author, the embarrassment cited by doctors (supposed or real) is taken into account in relation to private patients, as they are clients.

Although the patient in the public network needs to pay for the cost of drugs for hormonal hyperstimulation, as well as buying the inseminating dose (purchases necessary for specific procedures), which implies the ability to consume certain "goods", doctors do not take part in these transactions and do not make a profit from them, nor does their remuneration depend on the number of patients being treated. In contrast, in the private network, assisted reproduction appears as a service offered to a clientele with a certain consumption capacity. Doctors take part in the transactions and make a profit from them, as the costs of the treatment offered are paid directly by the client. In other words, the remuneration of these professionals depends on the number of patients/clients being treated. Hence, according to Costa, the concern about patients taking part in the research and the possible loss of clients.

Another study on the subject shows an advertisement for a private clinic specialising in conceptive reproductive technologies, located in the city of São Paulo, which offers plans from financial companies to pay for the treatments offered. According to Ramírez-Gálvez, the terms used in the advertising material are similar to those used by banks or credit institutions in their adverts, as can be seen in the following quote:

> At XXX, as well as having high technology and a specialised team, you also have instalment plans of up to 12 (twelve) payments, with or without a down payment through a financial institution. It's very easy. Simply complete the registration form and your dream of having a baby can come true. Note: subject to credit approval (RAMÍREZ-GÁLVEZ, 2002, p. 33).

This makes it clear that the dream of having a baby is treated in a similar way to the dream of owning a new car or a house of one's own, in other words, the child appears to be equated with the consumption of durable goods (RAMÍREZ-GÁLVEZ, 2002, p. 33).

According to Grossi et al. (2003), the discussion about assisted reproduction in Brazil points to the fact that the use of conceptive technologies is informed, among other things, by a logic of consumption. In this logic, assisted reproduction represents goods that can be purchased in pursuit of the ultimate goal, which is to have a child. This logic of consumption is what establishes different relationships between patients and doctors in private clinics and between patients and doctors in public clinics.

Marilyn Strathem (1992), likewise, analyses the advent of CTs within the framework of a consumer culture, based on the current so-called Western society. According to the author, in this consumer culture, value is placed on preference and choice in relation to consumer decision-making. And the prescription of consumption dictates that the consumer has no choice but to make choices according to their preferences; choices that are circumscribed by the goods offered by the market.

Strathern believes that those who seek assisted reproduction services are not thought of as patients looking for a remedy to cure their ailments, but as clients looking for services. Conceptive technologies enable people to fulfil desires that would not be realised without this help, provided they have the money. Choice, being a prerogative of consumption, is also the responsibility of the consumer, who must know how to choose what is best for them, according to their needs and preferences.

One factor that involves gamete donation from a consumer perspective is the way in which the material is acquired. As explained above, according to the rules of the Federal Council of Medicine, it is forbidden to trade in organs, tissues and gametes. However, the system to which human reproductive technologies belong seems to circumvent this prohibition, albeit indirectly, turning the practice of donation into a type of trade.

As explained in the first chapter of this thesis, in the case of semen, the purchase of the inseminating dose implies payment in cash to the supplier: the semen *bank,* even though the procedure is justified by the services involved in storing the material. Furthermore, the way in which donors are chosen is similar to the way in which goods are chosen for consumption. The characteristics of male gamete donors are presented to recipients by means of a list that resembles a "catalogue", where the consumer makes their choice. (COSTA, 2006, p. 3).

From the donor's point of view, although in Brazil the subject doesn't receive a financial reward, this does imply a return in terms of the laboratory and clinical tests offered by the semen bank, which the candidate/donor undergoes free of charge. It's worth pointing out that the same tests are carried out privately and involve high fees.

In the case of egg donation, as there are no female gamete banks, doctors resort to what they call *shared donation.* The term refers to the donation of eggs left over from patients undergoing IVF treatment in public hospitals to patients in private clinics, who share the costs of their treatment with the donors, since the medicines used in the public service are paid for by the patient, and are very expensive. (CORRÊA, 2001). In general, egg donors are younger women from less favoured social strata. Egg recipients, on the other hand, are generally older women from more favoured social strata. On the subject, it should also be emphasised that the *shared donation* system is only possible because most doctors working in the public sector have private clinics that offer assisted reproduction services (COSTA, 2006).

Still on the idea of consumer culture, it has to be considered that assisted reproduction arrived in Brazil almost exclusively through private medicine, a sector in which the vast majority of clinics and hospitals offering this type of service are still based today. The same happened with family planning information and methods (CORRÊA; LOYOLA, 1999). Reproductive technologies, both conceptive and contraceptive, although they can be found in the public service today, were introduced into the country by commercial interests, either from the pharmaceutical industry or from doctors.

This process of CT consumption also includes the issue of presenting the "product" as innocuous. According to Corrêa and Loyola, both the media and doctors publicise conceptive reproductive technologies in such a way as to make them seem simple, effective, accessible, harmless, capable of making up for nature's "deficiencies" and success rates are presented as high. However, according to the studies carried out by the researchers, these success rates are controversial. The following quote illustrates this:

> Because they have always been very low, it is well known that scientific circles have used the expedient of making up these rates in order to favour the apparent good *performance of* these techniques, [such a make-up consists of] choosing [for the calculation of the rate] categories that are favourable to the final result produced. (CORRÊA; LOYOLA, 1999, p. 219).

Costa (2006) suggests that the aspects observed in contacts with the different assisted reproduction services offered in the public and private sectors point to a lack of respect for ethical principles such as privacy and equality. The privacy of the identity of patients undergoing IVF treatment would be determined by their financial condition: according to their *status* as a patient in a public hospital or a client of a private clinic. On the other hand, semen and egg donation practices end up becoming commercial relationships masked by action strategies that circumvent the ban on the gamete trade.

At the same time, and paradoxically, the same technologies aimed at human reproduction are often allied with gestures of generosity, or with the notion of a gift, the subject of which will be discussed in the next section.

4.2 **Assisted reproduction: a question of gift?**

> [...] To give one's life is to transcend the mercantile experience defined as gaining one thing for the loss of another. Whoever gives their life not only loses nothing, since it is a gift-transmission, but also gains everything. They gain the fact that they give back the life they have been given without losing it and the possibility of giving it to someone for their entire life, someone who cannot be an object [...] (GODBOUT, 1999, p. 250).

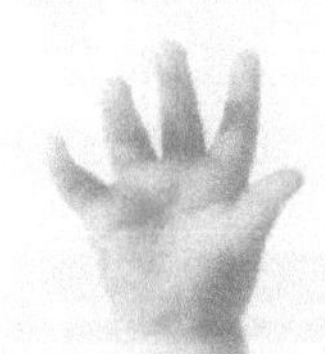

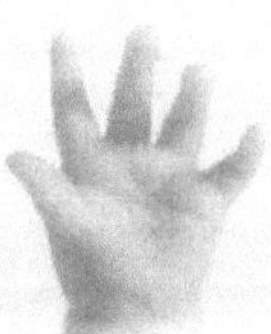

"Would you turn down a request for help like this?" is the phrase used at the opening of this *brochure* publicising Brazil's most significant semen bank. As you can see, at the ends of the sentence there is an image of two little baby hands, raised, as if they wanted to be held.

The message of the promotional material can be interpreted as a request for help to materialise a baby that only exists as a dream; a baby that is the focus of the actors who work with human reproductive technologies to achieve conception: the profession and science, the professionals, the users, the gamete donor, the surrogate mother and the body of techniques.

The *brochure* above covers various topics related to semen donation (the importance of paternity, the arrival of a child as the main factor in starting a family, prerequisites for donor candidates, guaranteeing identity secrecy, the legitimacy of the practice supported by current regulations, the credibility of the company providing the material, etc.), which are permeated by a strong appeal to an altruistic attitude, through which the donor is transformed into a "hero". The following quote is taken from the publicity material in question:

> Parenthood is one of the greatest emotions in a couple's life. [...] You can do a great deal of good in the lives of these couples. You can be their hope. Bring them closer to a dream [...]. It's a noble initiative that can bring untold happiness. Also for you, the donor. An action that will turn you into an unsung hero by helping to make a couple's life complete.

The appeal to altruism is frequent in the field of assisted reproduction and can be seen in most of the materials publicising the practice. The phenomenon is based on the fact that the desired result is the generation of human life. This aspect of the technique, combined with the alliances that are necessary to carry out the treatments, would promote the belonging of this medical speciality to the sphere of the gift. The professional dedicates his work to fulfilling other people's dreams of children; the techniques instrumentalise this fulfilment; the parents are the owners of the dream; the mother occupies a second place in the sphere of the gift, as the female gender. The semen donor and the egg donor provide their genetic material to a stranger in favour of the latter's desire. The surrogate mother temporarily donates her body for the pregnancy, in favour of forming a family that is foreign to her. The child is the main focus of the gift, representing the offspring, the dream, the gift itself, the one who will be given birth to.

The association of conceptive technologies with the sphere of the gift is commonly identified in the speeches of its actors. A doctor specialising in ART, who until then was a reference in the profession[19] , used the figure of God to justify the ethical and moral convenience of the practice, including embryo cloning, about which he was very optimistic. In an interview with the *São Paulo* newspaper *Folha de São Paulo,* he put the doctor in the place of a kind of divine emissary, who would be at the service of a good cause. Claiming to be a practising Catholic, the professional explained that:

> [...] everything is a question of the proper use of technology. Science in the service of a good cause is the closest thing to the materialist idea of divinity. For us, however, the presence of God, with his high designs, is what permanently guides the hands of scientists who seek to master the instigating phenomenon of conception. (ABDELMASSIH apud CORRÊA, 2001, p. 136).

Regarding the gift/surrogate motherhood dyad, we have the research of anthropologist Helena Ragoné, carried out between 1988 and 1990 in the United States. Her study looked at the three main actors involved in the practice: intermediary agencies, surrogate mothers and the couples who contract the services. It is worth noting that from the beginning of the field research, when artificial insemination prevailed as a treatment resource, to its conclusion, when IVF became a new option, assisted reproduction with egg donation increased from 5% (five per cent) to 50% (fifty per cent). At the same time, the proportion in which the gestational mother and the genetic mother were the same person fell from 95% (ninety-five per cent) to 50% [fifty per cent] (RAGONÉ, 1998, p. 196).

---

[19] Roger Abdelmassih was a prominent name in Brazilian assisted reproduction circles, as he was one of the pioneers in implementing the *IVF* method in the country. However, his *status* is currently under threat due to his involvement in crimes of rape, indecent assault and improper and illegal genetic manipulation. After numerous complaints from former patients, the doctor was arrested on 19 August 2009 and released on 24 December 2009 on a writ *of habeas corpus* granted by the president of the Federal Supreme Court (STF). Article available at: http://noticias.terra.com.br/brasil/noticias/0"OI4173904-EI5030,00-Abdelmassih+leaves+prison+after+habeas+granted+by+STF.html. Accessed on: 28/12/2009, at 20:2.

According to the results obtained by the researcher, the main philosophy of the surrogacy agency is to provide noble services, of extreme value to society, in terms of promoting contact between the two main parties in the treatment process: the surrogate mother and the creator(s) of the pregnancy. In addition, the agencies mediate legal issues, including contracts, and are committed to standardising the practice for those interested. Among their main guidelines is the avoidance of negative publicity for situations interpreted as immoral and exploitative. Because of this, the programmes usually limit their services to officially married heterosexuals, restricting access to the resource for single people and/or homosexual couples.

These agencies use newspaper adverts to recruit candidates for surrogacy, generally with themes that arouse altruistic feelings, similar to those identified in the semen donation material: "give the gift of life" and "help childless couples become a family". The policy of the agencies' programmes is to accept volunteers who are already mothers, both because it proves the woman's fertility and because it makes it easier to separate the baby after giving birth.

The women who offer themselves as surrogate mothers perceive the activity as a vocation and not as a simple service. In general, they are women who are already mothers, from the lower *Woorkni^* class, housewives, with traditional conceptions of the role of the female sex and the notion of the family. For them, the "gift of bearing a child" is an act that cannot be compensated financially, and the importance of remuneration is despised because it denigrates the image of selflessness associated with these mothers. Empathising with the suffering of infertile couples and the desire to experience pregnancy again without the burden of raising another child are admitted motivations for surrogacy.

Altruistic attitudes can also be seen among egg donors. For them, reproductive cells do not contain a physical reproductive capacity. They possess non-biological properties that are an effective way of helping others. These gifts would not be offered by them because they contain half of a genetic child, but rather because there is an expectation that the recipients will complete the development and care that the donors began. It would be a joint effort between donor and recipient to generate a new being, a child (LUNA, 2002).

According to studies on the subject, semen donation usually involves the varied and even contradictory factors of self-affirmation, pecuniary gain and altruism. The pecuniary nature of the practice is due to the feasibility of remuneration arising from the legislation of some countries, such as the United States (SALÉM, 1995). In the Brazilian case, as we have already seen, this possibility is vetoed. Altruism would exist in a similar way to that seen among other AR actors: helping infertile individuals and couples to realise the dream of parenthood, in favour of starting a family, whose baby is the target[20] . The aspects linked to self-affirmation would be reinforced by current Western sex and gender markers.

As we saw in the previous chapter, studies on the subject have pointed to the fact that the motivations for egg and semen donations seem to be inextricably linked to sex/gender issues: women are driven by altruism, while men are more focused on personal interests related to narcissism and the affirmation of male virility (HAIMES, 1993; YVON et al, 2004).

The child - generation and birth - occupies space in various dimensions of the gift: gift-birth, gift-sacrifice, gift-love, gift-life, gift-family, gift-transcendence, for whom all the other actors linked to conceptive reproductive technologies would be at the service, around whom this medical speciality revolves, the target of all gazes and actions, the beginning and end of the gift chain, situating the subjects in the incessant state of debt, which is linked to every gift. According to Jacques Godbout:

> It may seem strange that we make our relationship with our children a prototype of a gift relationship. But it's like that in many ways. First and foremost, birth is a gift. A gift of oneself par excellence, a gift of life, an original gift, motivating the gift relationship and the inclusion of all people in the state of debt, a debt from which the market and certain psychoanalysts want to free us. [...] The beginning of the gift chain lies there, for any individual, in a debt that they cannot assume except by giving their life in turn, which establishes the fundamentally non-dyadic, non symmetrical character of the gift. (GODBOUT, 1999, p. 5152).

Following the author,

> [...] the child is the being to whom we must give everything. Not only do we give them our lives, but they are also the only person for whom we spontaneously say that we are ready to give our lives. [...] The gift of a child is perhaps the most specific form of modern gift, and the debt incurred is the most difficult to assume. The child is the only person to whom modern society allows us to give without receiving. They are the God of modernity, the king, the one for whom everything can be sacrificed. With any other category of person, giving too much quickly becomes suspicious, strange, abnormal. The child is the only transcendence left (GODBOUT, 1999, p. 53).

In the Essay on the Gift, Mauss sought to demonstrate that the phenomena of the state and the market are not universal, since they can only be seen in more complex societies such as modern ones. However, in all societies that have existed in human

[20] According to the data collected in an interview with the management of a São Paulo sperm bank, altruism *is* perceived as the main motivating factor for sperm donation.

history - traditional or modern - it is possible to observe the constant presence of a system of interpersonal reciprocities, which expands or retracts based on a triple collective obligation to give, receive and return symbolic and material goods (MAUSS, 1974).

The author formulated a theory of the gift in which he systematised the complexity of exchange systems and the constitution of alliances. By defining society as a "total social fact", Mauss understood that social life is essentially a system of instalments and counter- instalments that oblige all members of the community, but not in an absolute way insofar as, in the concrete experience of social practices, the members of the community have a certain freedom to enter or leave the system of obligations - even if this can mean moving from peace to war. The gift introduces the idea of social action as "inter-action", as a circular movement triggered by the force of the good (symbolic or material) given, received and reciprocated, directly interfering both in the distribution of the places of the members of the social group, as well as in the modalities of recognition, inclusion and prestige.

The anti-utilitarian critique inspired by the tradition of Mauss aims to denounce the misunderstanding of any attempt to limit human motivations solely to the morality of interest and selfishness and to favour the market economy as the relevant instance in the production of social well-being. Mercantile logic would have a markedly predatory character when it is not under political and administrative regulation sanctioned by the community, proving that the aim of the market is not to generate social welfare, but the opposite, to produce profits, even if this means the end of jobs and.... social welfare. However, the social only arises under particular conditions of giving, trust and solidarity that cannot be explained from the perspective of individual interest or state bureaucracy, but from the paradox of the gift (GODBOUT; CAILLÉ apud MARTINS, 2005, p. 60).

> [...] The invention of the social only occurs through solidarity between individuals, in other words, through the risk of taking a spontaneous initiative to donate without guarantees of return and, equally, the risk of spontaneously accepting something from someone; this always uncertain and paradoxical initiative of giving, receiving and returning is known as the bet on the gift, a bet in which the value of the relationship itself is considered more relevant than the value of things or uses [...] (MARTINS, 2005, p. 60).

From the perspective of the gift, society and the individual are modes of manifestation of the *total social fact,* they are phenomenal possibilities that are incessantly engendered through a *continuum* of interrelationships motivated by the circulation of the "spirit of the thing given", or hau, these interdependencies unfolding between the various social spheres. Thus, according to Godbout (1999, p. 23) "(...) it is important to observe, as a priority in everyday life, not the actors and the structures, but what circulates between the actors in favour of the social bond": the material and symbolic goods that society has at its disposal in order to reproduce itself through the actors that make it up. The gift is present everywhere and does not only concern isolated and discontinuous moments in reality. What circulates has many names: money, cars, furniture, clothes, but also smiles, kindness, words, hospitality, gifts, free services, etc. For Mauss, what circulates has a decisive influence on how actors are formed and how their places in society are defined (MAUSS, 1974).

The perspective of the "gift paradigm" is that the founding rules of a society are essentially ambivalent and interdisciplinary. This logic proposes that there are rules specific to the economy, politics and the social sphere, but that society is only the result of the ambivalent way in which these different logics - irreducible to each other - take part in setting up the social game, but with the gift as the first and prior system to the others (which makes it the point of reference for a "gift paradigm"). Society is founded, above all, on the ambivalence of reciprocity: there is interest, but also disinterest, contract and spontaneous bond, paid and free.

Based on the above, we can think of the circulation of symbolic and material goods in heterologous ART as a system of gifts. The context of this technique contributes to the construction of the social, through its practices of solidarity between subjects - the bet on the gift - which is more relevant than the value of things or uses. Because it is the archaic logic that constitutes the social bond, the gift potentially integrates the possibilities of the market (retention of the donated good) and the state (possibilities of redistributing collective wealth), as seen in the medical speciality. The exchanges in question promote phenomenal possibilities through a *continuum* of interrelationships motivated by the circulation of the *haus* of the subjects involved; these interdependencies unfold between the various levels of society.

The following are some reflections on how reproductive practice is linked to the theory of the gift.

4.3 **Heterologous assisted reproduction as a system of gifts**

According to its characteristics, Jacques Godbout places both blood donation and organ donation in a mixed donation system, rather than a gift system
"pure". The same type of analysis can be extended to the donation of gametes. A mixed gift system is characterised as follows (GODBOUT, 1999, p. 107):

There is an importance of intermediaries between the donor and the recipient, and a particularly sophisticated technical-professional apparatus.

All these intermediaries, technicians and professionals are not governed by the gift, but by the wage relationship.

The technical-professional apparatus involved in the procedures in question is instrumental; it ensures the transmission of the gift.

Society does not accept the sale of donated "goods". The semen and egg trade is prohibited in Brazil.

According to the author, there is no doubt that the modern individual is constantly involved in gift relationships, but the modern gift represents an original form of circulation that is different from the one studied by both Mauss and most of the authors who study the subject and who reject gratuitousness. For Godbout, there are many differences between the gift and the commercial return. Firstly, *there is not always a return*, in the usual, mercantile sense of the term, of the material return of objects or services, as illustrated by the unilateral gift to strangers, taken in the sense of things that circulate. Secondly, conversely, *the return is often greater than the gift,* generally moving away from the principle of mercantile equivalence. Thirdly, *the return exists even if it wasn't desired.*

Giving has returns: the gratuity it gives rise to - the recognition - and that supplement that circulates and isn't included in the bill are important returns for the giver. Fourthly, *the return is often in the gift itself,* in the inspiration of the artist, and in the personal transformation undergone by those who give, for example. Those who do charitable work consider that they receive a lot from the people they help; they magnify themselves (GODBOUT, 1999, p. 113-115).

Mareei Mauss (1974), in the conclusion of his *Essay on the Gift,* suggests that a mixture of interest and gratuitousness characterises the majority of non-market exchange gestures in modern societies. Godbout (1999), who prioritises the gift as something of the order of the relationship, proposes that the inability to think of goods in the service of bonds leads to the suppression of all circulation of goods from affective bonds. This separation of the two watertight spheres can also be seen in everyday thinking. For many it is unacceptable, for example, to use commercial language (debt, exchange, payment) in the context of the gift, as is the case with paying money for the donation of gametes. Conversely, it's not a good idea to mix feelings with business (in which we can again include assisted reproduction). From a perspective in which all circulation of things is necessarily governed *only* by the principle of interest, this separation of the two spheres can be reached. In this sense, the mercantile model of society would have a double *status* - that of being one of the two, but also encompassing both, because even when we talk about the pure sphere of emotional bonds, where no goods should circulate, we tend to describe the bond as a good.

Godbout proposes a dissociation of the utilitarian and the gratuitous, so that modern thought *can* think of the two together, based on three types of value: *exchange value* (relating to the world of objects), *use value* (relating to service) and *bond value,* which is the value that any "gesture" has in the universe of bonds, in strengthening them, where the utilitarian-gift tension can be resolved. In addition to and independently of their exchange value and their use value, things have different values according to their ability to express, convey and nourish social bonds. However, this value is not established by comparison with other things, but above all in relation to people. "The same object has different bonding values depending on the circuit in which it is situated." (GODBOUT, 1999, p. 200). As for the gift, it has the capacity to enrich and transform the protagonists. The gift always contains an extra, a supplement, something more that gratuitousness tries to name: it is the value of the bond. The surplus value is the absorption of this supplement by the thing that circulates and by one of the protagonists, which is the transformation of a bond value into an exchange value. Bond value can be absorbed either by transforming it into use value, i.e. by interrupting the circulation of the thing and consuming it, or by objectifying it and reducing it to exchange value at the moment of making it circulate.

Link value is that which escapes calculation, which doesn't mean that it doesn't exist. Link value is the value of time, which the market replaces with an indefinitely extensible immediacy in space, removing the thing from the temporal network. The more things are isolated from their bond value, the more they become transportable, cold, frozen, pure objects that escape time. By expressing the value of the bond, the gift serves to prove to us that we are not objects. "Men who give confirm to each other that they are things". Thus we find the primitive gift and the *hau* of the Maori, as interpreted by Mauss, who defined it as the spirit of the thing that circulates. The thing that is given carries with it a bit of the person who gave it, which is nothing more than the value of the bond, or the symbolic exchange that is linked to the gift.

Focussing on CTs, and still following Godbout, the only gift ritual that can be compared, in both types of society (the so-called primitive and the so-called modern), is the one that accompanies marriage: birth and generation would effectively be the basis of any gift, whatever the society. Let's look at the quote below:

> Today, birth takes place in intimacy, in this protective enclosure invented by modern people against the dull world of production, which explains the displacement of the gift into this sphere of intimacy, which did not exist in primitive societies. The gift accompanies the birth and movement of life. The

> gift revolves around the family and kinship in both types of society. [...] (GODBOUT, 1999, p. 173).

However, for the author, the child born through human reproduction technologies may lead to the disappearance of this type of gift, since "these techniques are able to predict the sex of the child, its IQ, its genetic characteristics, etc., thus breaking the surprises of yesteryear." (Idem, p. 174). From this perspective, the conception of human life through AR may be transforming the baby who was in the absolute place of the gift into a product and birth into a production. Obviously, the birth that comes from heterologous assisted reproduction fits even more into this logic.

At various points in *The Spirit of the Gift,* Jacques Godbout is pessimistic about the existence of any kind of genuine gift in relation to the children "produced" by conceptive technologies. Similar concerns can be seen in academic discourse regarding the ethical issues involved in assisted reproduction practices, which include gamete donation. Not that these concerns aren't relevant; they very much are, but why not adopt another prism of the phenomenon, where it intersects with the gift? Because both the practice of donating gametes and the gift include bipolar rationalities, i.e. they can be analysed from the perspective of generosity or from the perspective of commerce. In scientific work, it's important to go beyond dichotomous thinking.

Procreation through assisted reproduction can be understood from a logic of commerce, thus damaging the notion of a genuine gift (if it exists), on the one hand, following Godbout. On the other hand, if we follow the same author's ideas about the value of the bond as a way of dissociating the utilitarian from the gift, we can understand the same type of procreation as being of the order of the gift, because, inevitably, bonds will be established between that child and those who live with it, bonds that will be built on a daily basis, just as happens in some cases.

cases, with the child born from sexual intercourse. I say "in some cases" because it would be naive to think that every child conceived naturally is the result of a genuine gift. To cite just one example, if the "natural" child is the result of a "belly flop" so that, through it, the mother is favoured with alimony, as a means of personal subsistence, such a conception would be based on a market logic, which would place it outside the notion of a genuine gift. Therefore, both modes of procreation - natural and artificial - can be equally inserted in the logics of gift and commerce. It is up to academic studies to better delineate the boundary that separates the two logics, thus guiding knowledge about the field that is emerging.

This research focussed on the theme developed in this chapter in order to broaden the reflections presented, based on an investigation into the factors that govern men's motivation to donate sperm at a Brazilian semen bank. The next chapter will present the field study carried out.

CHAPTER 5

THE FIELD STUDY

This chapter presents the field research carried out. I begin with the objective, followed by a presentation of the subjects recruited, the instrument used to collect the data, the procedures employed and the discussion and analysis of the material collected, ending with the results obtained.

5.1 **The research**

This study is characterised as qualitative research, based on a group of semen donors. Qualitative research can be characterised as an attempt to gain a detailed understanding of the meanings and situational characteristics presented by the sample, rather than producing quantitative measures of characteristics or behaviours. Qualitative methods tend to be unfavourable for measuring phenomena in large groups, but are useful for researchers seeking to understand the context in which a phenomenon occurs. They allow several elements to be observed simultaneously in a small group. This approach is capable of providing in-depth knowledge of an event, making it possible to explain behaviour (RICHARDSON et al, 1999, p. 90), which is congruent with the study carried out.

5.2 **Research strategies**

5.2.1 Objective

The aim of this study was to investigate men's motivation to donate gametes. This is a complementary procedure to CRTs, the process of which is entirely carried out by a semen bank: the recruitment of volunteers, the collection of material, laboratory procedures, up to the delivery of the inseminating dose to the recipient, which is mediated by previously registered professionals, clinics and/or hospitals in the field.

The focus of the study was on the factors that govern the desire of these individuals to donate semen to a specialised bank for the treatment of infertility cases of unknown people, since the practice is based on anonymity and gratuity.

5.2.2 Agents

The research was carried out with six male gamete donors registered at a semen bank located in the city of São Paulo.

The criterion used to recruit the study participants was that they wished to donate sperm to a Brazilian semen bank. Furthermore, individuals who had applied to the selection process and had not been accepted by the specialised clinic due to irregularities in the clinical examinations required of volunteers, as well as those who were still going through the selection phase at the bank, would have been included in the study. However, during the recruitment period, there was no demand from these groups of social actors.

The age range established for recruiting the subjects of this study followed the criteria adopted by the semen bank, but only in terms of the lower limit, since this is a group that is difficult to include. The study therefore selected men over the age of eighteen.

I would like to point out that data was collected on: education, profession, personal and family income, place of birth, nationality, place of residence (neighbourhood and city), marital status, number of children, if any, and race. However, this information was not considered a determining factor in selecting the subjects. They were only included as personal data and were used to support the analyses of the material collected in the investigation.

The number of interviewees in this research was not what was initially planned, but it was possible given the characteristics of the subject studied and the field in which the subject is inserted, which is characterised as difficult to enter. On this subject, I'm looking at the experience of Antonio Cândido who, although he didn't carry out exactly the same type of research as the one presented here, used a small group of "partners", as he put it, to find out about rural life in a group of caipiras from São Paulo. According to the researcher, the results obtained from the material collected, based mainly on individual cases, were satisfactory, based on the research proposal. According to the author:

> [...] the interest in individual cases, in significant details, is a fundamental element in this study, which was developed in the certainty that a sense of the qualitative is a condition for efficiency in the social disciplines, and that the sociologist's inner decision, developed through meditation and contact with the living reality of the groups, is as important as the technique of manipulating the data. It allows us to move from impression to hypothesis in many cases where the latter could not even be sketched according to statistical or accumulative criteria. (CÂNDIDO, 1987, p. 19).

Regarding his experience with the aforementioned research, demonstrating that the methodology used was favourable, Antonio Cândido says the following:

> [...] when I speak of the members of the group I studied, I am, at every moment, thinking of the caipira, in general; and, reciprocally, when I try to compose this methodologically useful abstraction, the real experience that proves it is, above all, that of the group I studied. (CÂNDIDO, 1987, p. 20-21).

In the case of the semen donor, as will be seen, from the six reports it was possible to find some answers to the question guiding this study: what motivates men to donate sperm to a specialised bank. It also revealed some clues about the field being researched. For, as anthropologist Ruth Cardoso states, the undeniable contribution of fieldwork as a way of understanding reality is "the presence of social actors, the supports of discourses, who have gained flesh and blood and are no longer automatons". (CARDOSO, 1986, p. 105).

5.2.2.1 Means of recruiting subjects

The subjects who took part in this research were recruited in three ways: through adverts published in a newspaper with a wide circulation in the state: *Folha de São Paulo*, and through contacts with a semen bank in São Paulo.

As far as the semen bank is concerned, posters publicising the research were put up on its premises, stating the type and purpose of the study and the contact details of the coordination team, and the same material was sent to the *emails* of around forty donors, taken from the clinic's database on two occasions. Due to the fact that only one candidate returned to the group, another thirty-five subjects were emailed, from which a further five responses were obtained. The documents sent the third time were:

a. Poster, as mentioned above.
b. Free and informed consent form.
c. Notice to donors.

The *notice to donors* was a piece of material drawn up in mid-2009 with the aim of sensitising individuals to take part in the research by providing details about the importance of scientific studies for the construction of knowledge, together with detailed information about the research in question and its coordinator.

The newspaper was published in *Folha de São Paulo* for three days in October 2009 (Saturday, Tuesday and Thursday) and, for a period of thirty days, in its *online* format - *Folha Online.* From these mass media outlets, there were only four returns, which were summarised as curious men looking for information on the subject of sperm donation. They were referred to the semen bank with which the research had contact at the time.

5.2.3 Locations where fieldwork was carried out

The fieldwork carried out with the semen donors took place in the municipalities of São Paulo and Rio de Janeiro.

Since all the agents live in São Paulo, it was more convenient for the group to hold the meetings there. So the researcher travelled to the capital of São Paulo to carry out the practical part of the investigation, which took place in June and November 2009. During this period, on a bank holiday, one of the subjects travelled to Rio de Janeiro and took the opportunity to schedule an interview. As the event took place on a Sunday evening, the venue used was the study coordinator's home. As for the other meetings, it's worth noting that while conducting the field study in São Paulo was favourable for the agents, it also made the research more difficult.

As all the interviews were recorded and the data collected is always confidential, especially when the subject is a practice that involves anonymity, the physical space to receive the subjects required silence and privacy, which became an important difficulty to overcome, due to the fact that the researcher does not live in the city of São Paulo. This reality implied a number of limitations: the doctoral student's circle of interpersonal relationships (professional, family and friends) is much smaller there than where she lives, the capital of Rio de Janeiro. Knowing a large number of people increases the chances of favours being provided, such as the loan of premises to conduct the investigation, for example, or even the provision of tips on suitable places for this type of meeting, among others. In addition, the lack of familiarity with the municipality and the lack of knowledge about the characteristics of its neighbourhoods, shops, distances and transport, made travelling extremely difficult, minimising the possibilities of areas that could be used for interviews.

In addition to these factors, there was also the need to reconcile the research coordinator's time on site with the always scarce time of the also scarce donors willing to contribute to the research, which ended up requiring the use of weekends as meeting opportunities, when, on the other hand, most of the commercial establishments were closed. Finally, as well as having to adjust the schedules of the researcher and all five interviewees, the former's time in the municipality had to be very limited due to economic factors, as a doctorate-level study generally does not have large financial resources.

In this sense, several contacts were made in order to find the ideal place to meet the research subjects. At this stage we relied on referrals from the research supervisor, professional colleagues and friends, as well as strangers from Rio de Janeiro and São Paulo, as well as internet searches.

Since the beginning of 2009, when the programme to carry out the practical part of the study began, numerous locations were contacted. These included: the vice-rector of the Department of Preventive Health at UNIFESP, part of the Federal University of São Paulo; the directorate, secretariat and library of the Faculty of Public Health at the same university; the directorate of the CRM-SP - São Paulo Regional Medical Council; the directorate of the CRP-SP - São Paulo Regional Psychology Council. All the institutions mentioned were approached via telephone calls and email, when requests for space were made.

As instructed by the institutions they had contacted, *emails* were sent after the phone calls with the following attachments: a summary of the research project, details of the characteristics of the room to be used and the dates and times for its use. Only the CRP got back in touch, offering to provide a room to host the study. At the time of the planned trip to São Paulo, three *emails* were sent to the department responsible to confirm that the space would be provided. Only the last one was returned, when the Council's management cancelled the offer on the grounds that there would be a class event on the scheduled date. It is worth pointing out that the applicant had already been invited to the Council for a large regional congress, which was also attended by the Federal Council of Psychology and several Brazilian researchers. The CRP-SP headquarters building is large, with several floors, rooms and a modern auditorium which, even at the event mentioned, in 2003, didn't even occupy 1/3 (one third) of the total area. This raises different possibilities to those put forward by the Council. On the other hand, it is interesting to note that all the other contacts remain unanswered to date.

Due to the difficulties encountered in finding a place to receive the agents, other possibilities were considered, such as the premises of a hotel or subletting a few hours at a psychologist's office. Therefore, the locations for data collection were chosen in line with the donors' preferences. The first two meetings took place in a building called *Conjunto Nacional,* on Paulista Avenue in the south of São Paulo: one in the café of a bookshop and the other on the terrace. The final three interviews took place in the room of a hotel in the República neighbourhood, where the researcher stayed, as part of the group could only make it on Friday and the other part on Saturday.

5.3 Research limitations

There are endless ways to develop scientific methodologies and all of their stages must be in line with the configuration of the study: the way in which the object of study was delimited, its general and specific objectives, among others, always taking into account the advantages and disadvantages that each element of the research strategies can introduce to the research. This study's methodology was drawn up along these lines, as well as being consistent with the analyses that follow:

> "[...] social research techniques cannot be used as recipes or neutral instruments, but as means of obtaining information whose qualities and limitations must be controlled," because in this type of research the social object is man and subjectivities are at play throughout the research process (RICHARDSON et. al., 1999, p. 219).

5.3.1 Instruments used for data collection

> The best situation for participating in the mind of another human being is face-to-face interaction, because it has the unquestionable character of proximity between people, which provides the best possibilities for penetrating the mind, life and definition of individuals (RICHARDSON et al., 1999, p. 207).

Guided by the notions of Roberto Richardson mentioned above, this research chose the interview technique as the instrument through which the data for this study was collected. This instrument can be defined as a technique in which the investigator presents himself to the person being investigated and asks them questions, with the aim of obtaining the data that is of interest to the investigation. The interview is therefore "a form of social interaction. More specifically, it is a form of asymmetrical dialogue in which one party seeks to collect data and the other presents itself as a source of information." (GIL, 1999, p. 117).

> As a data collection technique, the interview is very suitable for obtaining information about what people know, believe, expect, feel or want, intend to do, do or have done, as well as their explanations or reasons for the above (SELLTIZ et al. apud GIL, 1999, p. 117).

In order to collect statements from the subjects of this study, semi-structured interviews were carried out individually. These are characterised by the use of a script whose function is to guide the meeting between researcher and researched.

The script used in this study[21] - being semi-structured - was made up of two parts: the first (structured) contains the well-defined questions, the identification data, and the second, the topics that were covered in the interview. As an example of one of these, I chose the item "Experience with sperm donation at a semen bank". This item was presented as a topic and not as a question. Thus, in each interview the questions were formulated in a different way and presented at different times to each subject, depending on the flow of the dialogue. Thus, if the interviewee spontaneously anticipated their answer to a question planned for the future, the interviewer could stop repeating it, addressing what was asked at the exact moment. This is a "flexibility" in conducting the interview, so that a relaxed atmosphere is favoured, which can have a positive impact on the researcher-interviewee interaction, as was seen in the data collection stage of this research. However, it should be emphasised that in this type of instrument, it is essential that all the items in the semi-structured part are included in all the interviews.

The script used in this research was tested in the first two interviews. As the instrument did not require any adjustments, it was considered suitable for the final applications. The preliminary meetings were therefore included in the final material.

---

[21] The script can be found in the annexes to this thesis.

Finally, it is important to point out that the choice of this data collection instrument was due to the depth that is considered possible when using interviews, which was in line with both what was idealised and what was experienced during the field study stage.

The topic that guided this study was the *motivation for donating one's own genetic material to unknown people and to a semen bank, with* the act being based on the rules of gratuitousness and anonymity of the identities of the individuals involved in the process [donors, parents who conceived the pregnancy and the child].

On a second level, we investigated whether the factors motivating semen donation are related to characteristics of the practice, such as anonymity, gratuitousness, among others, as well as whether they are associated with other aspects, such as Western notions of family, kinship, etc. The procedure sought to obtain answers to the phenomenon in question. In this sense, in addition to the topic of motivation for semen donation, other elements were raised, which will be presented in the data analysis.

5.2.6 Procedures

As mentioned above, as the script was judged to be satisfactory when the first two interviews were carried out, they were added to the final research material.

A total of six individual interviews were carried out in locations selected by mutual agreement between the subjects and the interviewer, as explained in subsection 5.2.3 above.

All the meetings were recorded on a Panasonic digital mini-recorder, model RR-US450. Unlike the old mechanisms, in which cassette tapes were still used, this device makes it possible to: record the sounds in high resolution; count the time spent at the event in hours, minutes and seconds; transfer the digitised data to CD/DVD media or to the computer's memory; and it has uninterrupted operation.

The characteristics of the recorder used in this field study meant that the quality of the two interviews was not jeopardised, given that they took place in public places where there was a lot of noise.

Once the data collection stage was complete, all the material was transcribed in full and recorded in *Word* programmes. The interviews were then printed out and prepared for the analysis phase.

5.2.7 Analysing the data

The material collected using the structured interview methodology is qualitative in nature, which implies the need to analyse the data qualitatively, the treatment of which involves a set of procedures aimed at organising them in such a way that they reveal, as objectively and impartially as possible, how the research subjects perceive and relate to the focus of the study in question (IERVOLINO; PELICIONI, 2001).

A number of procedures were used to carry out the analysis. Firstly, after each contact with the field through the interviews, the researcher's perceptions of each meeting were recorded. Subsequently, each statement was listened to and transcribed into a *Word* document, the final product of which was kept in a specific database, following the coordinator's records, and in date order, based on the day the interviews took place.

Transcribing the data collected always requires more time than applying the collection instruments, which can be seen as a labour-intensive stage, but one that is of paramount importance for the research, as it allows each interview to be studied, proceeding with a preliminary analysis of the results achieved. (RICHARDSON et. al, 1999, p. 217-218).

After the transcriptions, the material was processed and analysed according to the technique of content analysis, which emphasises the description of how certain explanatory categories appear or are absent from the discussions, and in which contexts this occurs, in order to better configure the aspects or topics, and the categories on which the analyses will be based, since such material is important for defining the categories themselves (BARDIN, 1970).

In qualitative research, unlike quantitative research, the frequency of a characteristic is less important than its presence (or absence) for the essential meanings of the message to be extracted. This study used the mixed model, in which the categories are selected prior to data collection, but with the flexibility for possible changes depending on the analysis. This research model is not limited to checking for the presence of predetermined elements; all elements that prove to be significant are considered, even if the researcher has to expand the field of categories or eliminate some.

In the analysis stage, the first step is to immerse the researcher in the data collected by reading all the material obtained. The next step is to write down the qualitative categories that will be highlighted as most important, based on this first systemic contact with the material being analysed. After a constant review of the data, the main categories are chosen, which are created according to recurring responses from the interviewees.

After transcribing the meetings and printing out the material, a general reading was made of each interview, mapping out what the interviewees had said in relation to each topic in the script. At this point, the issues discussed were highlighted throughout the texts. In *Bardin*'s *discourse analysis* technique, this stage is called *floating reading.*

So, let's suppose that the topic of "religion" was mentioned by the interviewee on pages two, five and ten. Next to their respective paragraphs, the subject under discussion is highlighted.

This moment is called intra-subject analysis, when each interview is analysed individually and possible inconsistencies or contradictions in each agent's discourse are looked for. An example of this would be someone saying they don't intend to have children and then revealing that they spend hours thinking about the day they become a father. When these contradictions or inconsistencies were found, there was yet another stage, which was to see if there were similar contradictions/inconsistencies in the statements of the other subjects.

At this stage of the work, all the individually analysed material had already been grouped in terms of its classification and for each of the interviewees, so we moved on to the next stage: inter-subject analysis. The essential thing in this part of the analysis is to have an overview of the material, reading it across the board, i.e. looking for how a particular theme appears in each interview. To do this, a table was created for each subject broken down into topics in the script. Thus, a table was built for *knowledge of the topic,* another table for *the approach to the practice of semen donation,* another for *experience with semen donation,* and so on. In each of the tables, the data from all the subjects was grouped together, which had already been previously categorised by topic.

The next phase consisted of writing up the results obtained, which will be presented later in section 5.3, which refers to the discussion and analysis of the research data.

It should be noted that the process of analysis often takes place simultaneously with data collection. In addition, all the material obtained is understood as a source of analysis: the researcher's perception of the field, now recorded; the way in which contacts took place prior to the face-to-face meeting, usually via *email* or telephone; the type of bond established between researcher and deponent; the textual quotes from the subjects, which may illustrate the main findings of the analysis, among others. Since it adopts a process in which categories and explanatory hypotheses are formed from the data, it is standard procedure in qualitative research to reflect on and analyse the partial results, with a view to better adapting the data collection procedures to the research objectives.

Before moving on to the section on the discussion and analysis of the research data, we will explain the approval process for this study with the Human Research Ethics Committee, which was an important stage in carrying out the fieldwork.

5.2.8 The Human Research Ethics Committee

From the 19th century onwards, the practice of medicine became linked to scientific research and living, healthy human beings began to be subjected to its methods and procedures for validation and justification. In ethical terms, the principle of the researcher's good intentions was enough for research to be morally justified. With the double paradigmatic transition in science and ethics, based on historical and cultural factors (technological development, the counter-culture movement, etc.), the principles of autonomy and equity were associated with the old principles of non-maleficence and beneficence - the only ones governing the medical act until then - and began to guide decisions regarding scientific practices, with the aim of curbing the growing practice of abuses against human subjects, previously justified by an apparent scientific interest (SCHRAMM et al., 2008).

Nowadays, this model forms the basis of many resolutions and guidelines on the ethical conditions necessary for research involving human beings, such as Brazilian Resolution no. 196/96 and the complementary regulations of the CNS (National Health Council)[22] , which is linked to the Ministry of Health and to which the Brazilian Research Ethics Committees are subordinated.

The CEP (Research Ethics Committee) is the institutional body accredited by CONEP (National Commission for Ethics in Research)[23] , linked to the CNS, which aims to protect the well-being of research subjects. It is an interdisciplinary committee, made up of professionals of both sexes, as well as at least one representative from the community, whose role to analyse, assess and monitor research projects that involve the participation of human beings, with regard to the ethical issues involved. The IMS (Institute of Social Medicine) at UERJ (Rio de Janeiro State University), where this study is being carried out, has had a Research Ethics Committee, the CEP-IMS, since 2000 .[24]

Initially, on 23/03/2009, this research project and the researcher responsible for the investigation were registered with SISNEP (National Information System on Ethics in Research Involving Human Beings)[25] , which generated a document called a "cover sheet", which was given the registration number FR-249997. Subsequently, on 27/03/2009, the process formed for the present investigation was forwarded to the CEP-IMS, and was approved at a meeting held on 14/05/2009, under CAAE - 0009.0.259.000-09, based on the declaration of the same date of the meeting, signed by Maria Helena

[22] For more information, go to: *http*://conselho.saude.gov.br.
[23] For more information, go to: *http://conselho.saude.gov.br/comissao/eticapesq.htm.*
[24] For more information, go to *http://www.ims.uerj. br/cep.*
[25] For more information, go to: http://portal2.saude.gov.br/sisnep/pesquisador.

Costa-Couto. The following documents were included in the CEP-IMS review request process:

F SISNEP *cover sheet.*

b. *Research protocol,* in which project data was entered: title; names and addresses to access the *lattes* CVs of the researcher responsible, the supervisor and the co-supervisor of the study; abstract; subject area; methodology; provision for interrupting the study (if this had been the case); critical analysis of the risks and benefits of the research; expected results; statement of the resources and costs involved in carrying out the field research; guarantee of confidentiality of the information collected and the main bibliographical references (two copies).
c. The *script* that served as a guide for the field research (two copies).
d. Free and informed *consent form* (two copies).
e. *Declarations* of responsibility regarding: the publication of the results obtained; the coordinator's responsibility and confidentiality regarding the use and destination of the material and data collected; the commitment to comply with CONEP Resolution no. 196/96 and the protocol statements (two copies).
f. Research execution *schedule* (two copies).
g. *CV of* the researcher responsible for the study (two copies).
h. *Media* (CD) on which the documents presented here were saved.

5.3 Presentation of the discussion and analysis of the data obtained

According to the data obtained from the interviews, all the interviewees donated semen to a specialised bank, due to factors related to the sphere of gift. However, based on the testimonies, each of the six subjects was linked to the sphere of the gift in a very unique way. In other words, the desire that mobilised them to donate has close links to the gift, and the impetus for the act was shaped by their life stories, experiences, expectations, the way they have constructed themselves as people, among other things. This being the case, it seemed more appropriate to reconstitute these characters, putting together a "portrait" of each of them, with the aim of presenting them and bringing the reader the real "encounters" that resulted from the field study.

In most of the "encounters", as the interviews unfolded, the investigated, in alliance with the researcher, both made their points and realised issues they had never thought of before, which produced real discoveries on both sides about the field studied, as well as a range of emotions filled with laughter and tears. Right,

> The intersubjective relationship is not a meeting of autonomous and self-sufficient individuals. It is a symbolic communication that presupposes and restores basic processes responsible for creating meanings and groups. It is in this encounter between people who are strangers and who move closer together

> that can uncover hidden meanings and make unknown relationships explicit (CARDOSO, 1986, p. 103).

One caveat should be made here. Although the phenomenon of the "encounter" belongs to the sphere of the gift and some authors place great value on the subject, such as *Fritz Pearls*, creator of the *gestalt* psychotherapeutic approach, who prioritises contact as the main tool for behavioural change, and sociologist *Randal Collins,* who continued an interesting theory started by *Durkheim* that analyses human relationships based on the idea of *emotional energy,* which refers to a special type of energy that varies depending on the type of ritual the individual is part of, this research is not based on these themes. The intention was simply to emphasise how rich the interviews were, which, rather than being instruments for collecting research data, produced real "encounters".

This section will present the paths taken by the subjects towards understanding what moved them to the practice of semen donation, interpreted by them as a "life goal", or even a "mission", as an "urgency", or an "exchange of favours", which became the main category of this study.

5.3.1 Entering the field: getting to know the semen bank

My introduction to the field of reproductive technologies began in the second half of 2006. At that time, the object of study was still being circumscribed, but semen donation had already been chosen as the subject of the thesis. As such, an exploratory search on the internet identified around three clinics specialising in the cryopreservation of male gametes, the most representative of which was located at the *Albert Einstein Hospital,* as already mentioned in sub-section 1.2.1. Once I had the data, I made telephone contact with the management of the semen bank, who were informed about the research, its institutional links and asked for support in the process of recruiting the target audience. On the grounds that the group to be studied would not agree to be approached, the answer received was negative.

Two years later, when the field work was beginning to be defined, new contact was made with the semen bank. However, at that time it was located in its own premises. In a conversation with the company's management, the subject of the research was discussed, after which a date was requested to make face-to-face contact with the bank. The meeting took place a week later.

I arrived at Avenida Paulista at half past eight in the morning and immediately spotted the cross street , where the semen bank is located. It's on the ground floor of a modern, showy commercial building. After passing a guardhouse at the end of the pavement, I identified the entrance to the clinic by its logo. I announced myself over the intercom and was told to go in and wait at reception. Taking the entrance door as a reference, on the right hand side there is a small window that allows you to contact a bank employee. On the left there are stairs and a toilet.

The room is finely decorated with colourful walls, two light armchairs with a bold *design*, a sideboard *with folders* advertising the venue, beautiful pictures on the walls, magazine racks with a variety of current issues, and some decorative pieces in the style of the venue. Everything inspired modernity, refinement, good taste, discretion and silence. Apart from the member of staff standing beyond the little window, who never appeared again, I only saw someone else when the director, Simone, arrived[26] , whom I was waiting for.

When she walked through the door and saw me at reception, Simone introduced herself in a very courteous manner and immediately directed me to the second floor of the clinic, where her office is located. We went up a white staircase and entered a room similar in appearance to that of a doctor's surgery, with a table, a chair on one side (clinician) and two on the other (patient), as well as a stretcher for examination. Unlike the first floor, the whole of the second floor is white, which perhaps makes everything there seem a little invisible.

Simone and I discussed the research in progress, its objectives and the need to have the support of the semen bank to publicise the study. The directorate was presented with the documentation proving my institutional affiliation, the supervisor's endorsement, the approval of the research by the Ethics Committee, the CEP-IMS, as well as the draft of the material to be used in the donor recruitment stage. I also took advantage of the meeting to record an interview in order to gather data on the field. Simone was helpful, making herself available to help with the subsequent phase of the research, agreeing to put up posters inside the clinic and also sending them to the *emails of* some of the men in the company's database. After our meeting, the director accompanied me to the exit door on the first floor, where we said a fond farewell.

As soon as the poster was printed, I sent a reasonable amount to the semen bank by post and a few weeks later, Milton Jardim sent a message to the research email address. We corresponded a few times and, with the aim of receiving more applicants, I asked the subject to wait for future contact. After a month, no further *emails* had arrived. So I contacted Simone again, asking her to kindly send the material to new donors, which she promptly did.

Two more months passed and no other candidates for participation in the research

[26] As already mentioned in the Alíscia Baensi case, all the first names of the participants in this research are fictitious.

came forward. So I decided to contact the semen bank again. I was informed that the poster had been fixed to the reception desk and sent to the *emails of* several individuals, around 40 (forty). As the response was minimal, I decided to reformulate the way I approached the class. I wrote a "notice to donors", in which I explained the aims of the proposed research, the approval of the research protocol by the Ethics Committee, the difficulties I was encountering in getting the group studied to take part in the research, and the importance of scientific studies for the construction of knowledge. In addition, personal and professional details were mentioned, as well as the *emails* and telephone numbers of the research coordinator, with the aim of realising communication between the parties. A dramatic tone was deliberately used in the document in question to sensitise those who had access to the material. In order to inspire greater confidence in the subjects, I decided to add the free and informed consent form to the publicity material, which gives guarantees to the research subject and the research.

With this new strategy in place, I phoned the bank and was, as always, kindly answered by the management when I informed them of the change in the way I approached the subjects. I explained the urgency in which I found myself, due to the short time I had left to complete my doctorate, taking into account all the stages I still had to go through: qualification, field study, completion of the thesis and the defence of the work. I was fully aware that I was being insistent, as she is an extremely busy professional, and I apologised with every phone call, but once again I asked for the current dossier (poster, press release and terms of reference) to be sent to the donors in order to recruit the target audience, to which the coordinator agreed. Not only was the material sent, but it was addressed to each of the twenty men with the following message:

> *"Paulo, I'm sending you this email to see if it's possible for you to take part in some research by Ana Paula into semen donation. The main theme of the research is the motivation for donation, in other words, what factors are involved in the act of donating, based on which man decides to donate semen.*
>
> *The publicity poster and consent form are attached. If you can help, please contact Ana Paula directly. Email: .pesquisa_doacao@ims.uerj.br*
>
> *Thank you,*
>
> *Simone P.S. "*

Immediately after my message was forwarded, I received another contact. At that point, it totalled two.

I perceived the field as barren and decided to go to São Paulo before I missed these two precious research opportunities. The "encounters" we had with the six semen donors we interviewed in this study are presented below.

The main aim of inserting this part into the thesis was to provide the reader with the most relevant elements that characterised each encounter with each semen donor, as a way of presenting the agents of the phenomenon being researched.

5.3.2 Composing "portraits" or "encounters" with semen donors

First meeting: **Milton Jardim**

Milton Jardim is twenty-eight years old, has a law degree, works professionally as a federal civil servant, has a monthly income of R$4,000.00 (four thousand reais) and a family income of R$6,500.00 (six thousand five hundred reais), is married, has no children, lives in the Higienópolis neighbourhood of the city of São José do Rio Preto, considers himself Catholic, classifies himself as white, and has been donating semen for a year.

The agent was the first donor to contact the research email address. He had been waiting for the interview date for four months, and from the start he was very keen to give his testimony. The initial contacts were all by *email* and, as we got closer to our meeting, we started talking on our mobile phones.

At his suggestion, the interview took place in the café of *Livraria Cultura* do *Conjunto Nacional,* located on Avenida Paulista, in the south of São Paulo, early in the morning, at 8.30am on a Saturday. As well as enjoying getting up early, on this day and time the place is pretty empty, which changes configuration as time goes by.

As far as I was concerned, I managed to get to the metro that would take me to the scheduled stop at eight hours and fifteen minutes, and I had no idea how long it would take me to reach my destination. I decided to make a phone call to warn the chap about a possible delay. Milton answered promptly: "I'm already here at the café and it's no problem if you're late. I'll wait as long as it takes. Don't worry. I was relieved when he returned. At the same time, it was clear how willing he was to talk.

When I arrived at our meeting point in the café, I saw several tables, about twenty-five, and a few armchairs on the sides of the room, where customers could sit and read some of the bookshop's products. Some tables were occupied, but I soon identified my subject. He was a young man, of medium build, handsome and well-dressed in a classic style. I approached him, we identified ourselves and after a trivial chat and a cup of coffee, which had *the* function of a *rapport* establishment[27] , we began the interview.

He begins his speech with the first topic of the script: "I knew there was such a thing as semen donation, but I didn't know how it was done or anything". When he decided to donate semen, Milton had little knowledge of the world. The desire emerged from him, regardless of any publicising of the practice, or any other reason.

To get information on the subject, she turned to the *Google* search engine on the internet, where she found the semen bank that operated on the premises of the *Albert Einstein Hospital.* The distance between the clinic and his work, coupled with limited time available, prevented him from realising his intention at the time. A year later, the desire to become a semen donor resurfaced. Again, he turned to the same search engine, where he found the previous bank in a new location, now close to the public office where he works. He immediately made contact by telephone, booked an appointment and turned up on the scheduled date, already in a state of sexual abstinence, as instructed by the clinic. Once there, he had a consultation, tests, semen collection, asked all his questions and, after the quarantine period, was accepted as a donor by the bank.

The factors that motivated Milton to donate semen were not evident at the beginning of the interview, but they emerged in parts. Investigating his story gave me an impression that resembled putting together a jigsaw puzzle. At first, the inconsistencies, incoherencies, gaps and unanswered whys revealed an obscure point. When I questioned him, he would say things like: "Ah, good question! I don't think I can answer you". On several occasions, the best option was to leave the question on *standby* while we focussed on another topic in the interview script.

Milton reported that the main reason that led him to become a semen donor was the desire to have many children, which could perhaps be explained by his childhood experience. He and a sister were brought up by their mother, as the parents separated when the children were very young and the father became absent. As his mother was of Italian descent and the family tradition with this ancestry is usually a strong alliance between family members, the interviewee says he grew up with his cousins, uncles and grandmother. According to him:

> I grew up with my cousins. With my sister, there were five of us. We grew up together and our uncles were there too. So we were very close, everyone at grandma's house on Sundays. I think the fact that I was brought up with a lot of people around may have unconsciously influenced my desire for many

[27] The American Heritage dictionary defines rapport as "A relationship, especially one of mutual trust or emotional affinity". In other words, to establish good rapport is to create bonds of affinity, which is very important at the start of an alliance, whether at a professional or private level.

children, I don't know. (Milton)

As the understanding of "many children" has varied over time in so-called western societies, I asked Milton about his understanding of "many children", to which he replied: five. At first it was clear that the number of children he wanted coincided with the number of children he had in his childhood group, but it didn't make much sense with his *desire to donate semen.* For the time being, I opted to take another route, putting my thinking on temporary hold. The focus shifted towards the feasibility of the interviewee having the number of children he wanted in "real life", since his intention could be fulfilled in marriage to his wife, or even outside the marriage covenant, with different women. Thus, semen donation would not be necessary. The difference between one path and the other lay in the possibility of contact with descendants, which would be anonymous in the latter case.

Milton reports that his wife accepts having up to two children. According to him: "She says that two children are a good size, and that when the first one is born, I'll give up on wanting a second one". As for the idea of being a father with different wives, he doesn't see the possibility because he lives in a monogamous society. His situation would not be accepted. However, even though he realises that he wouldn't have social approval to have children with different women, at this point he exposes a desire that has been with him for a long time: to have children with ethnically diverse women, which still doesn't seem to answer the research question.

> I didn't stop to think about it, but one thing I even said to my wife, if I wasn't going to get married and have children, I would, let's say, be curious to have one with each type of woman: an Asian, a black, a white, an Indian, just to see what the children would be like. This could be one of the answers, but when I decided to donate, I didn't think about it. I simply wanted to be a donor. (Milton)

Let's return to the initial point: their motivation for donating semen. The desire to have many children appears to be the main reason for the act, but there is another point. In his words: "If I couldn't have (a child), I'd like my wife to have one. I'd like her to be able to use a semen bank to get pregnant". This new motive could be "dissected" into two parts. Was sperm donation idealised to help those who experience what, in the donor's fantasy, could happen in their own marriage, or was the deponent making a kind of "saving" of his reproductive cells, which could serve the couple in the event of them becoming sterile?

Milton doesn't share either of these thoughts, he just likes the idea of there being a semen bank where his wife could get pregnant in the event of his hypothetical sterility. On the other hand, he has never made donations with the idea of helping someone else in mind, but rather prioritised his own reasons: himself and his wife. Still, according to the interviewee, "if someone is in the same situation, they go and get it". Based on this statement, I asked him if he was thinking of someone other than himself and his wife. Milton agrees and concludes: "I thought directly about his wife and, indirectly, I thought about other people".

We already had some pieces of the puzzle, but the whole was not complete. We had to keep digging deeper, investigating. Why would Milton have decided to become a semen donor, driven by what idea, by what feeling? This point of the main research question was still unclear.

We return to the initial question. Milton says that he donated semen because he wants to have lots of children and that he was thinking of his wife, as mentioned above. We took a different route. As of that date, seven donations had been made. I proposed a "journey" aimed at associating the desire for many children with his satisfaction, based on the children that come from the donation. I ask him to imagine that he has learnt that his seven donations have already been used by recipients, generating seven pregnancies, seven births and, finally, seven babies who are his biological children. I ask him if his desire to have many children has been fulfilled. For Milton, these children are desired, but as he won't be aware of their existence, he explains: "I think it will be indifferent, because the children are anonymous". I say that if he wants these children, even if they are anonymous, they must symbolise something in his life. He agrees, but doesn't know how to answer this question. According to the interviewee: "Now I don't know how to answer it, I can't answer it".

Trying to untangle the "knot" that had been left, Milton presents three alternatives that would justify his motivation for donating semen:

1. As the society in which he lives is monogamous, and the alternative of producing children with different women would not be accepted, his offspring via donated semen would be a way of having the many children he wants.
2. His Christian (Catholic) background, with which he has an affinity.
3. The curiosity of having different children, because they would be born to different women.

These justifications, in my opinion, produced new "knots" instead of clarifying the previous obscurity. The first issue was contradicted in relation to the other discourse, when he revealed that the children generated through the donation would not fulfil his desire for many children, because they were anonymous. His Catholic upbringing didn't seem to justify the donation. If the Catholic Church's views are usually based on family traditions and conservatism, how could that religious strand and semen donation be related? Finally, how would his curiosity about ethnically different children be realised if he didn't even know they existed?

Once again, I chose to leave the data in abeyance until it made sense. We return to the "journey" we proposed earlier: the meaning of the children who supposedly exist from semen donation. For Milton, these children represent self-perpetuation. According to the interviewee, "We came here to.... came here to live, of course! Everything But it's the natural cycle of life: you're going to have children and so on.
continuing". I questioned the fact that your perpetuation will be resolved when the child you have with your wife is born, which is about to happen any day now, according to your information.

I reworked his entire line of reasoning, showing the inconsistencies that had arisen. Disconnected pieces of the "jigsaw" were being provided and there would come a time when they would make sense, when they were clear, when they were put together. At this point, the interviewee talks again about his desire to perpetuate himself, but now it would be because he really enjoyed his childhood: living with his family, the atmosphere of his grandmother's house, etc.

I ask him if a woman "agreed" to have five children with him, would she still donate semen? He replies: "I've already donated. I wouldn't try to stop it, to withdraw the donation, but it's a good question". I mention the possibility that this agreement occurred before he became a donor, to which he replies: "I think I would continue to donate... I would."

Since, in the imaginary situation, his desire for many children and self-perpetuation would have been fulfilled, what factor would still be governing his desire to be a semen donor? Milton reflects for some time and concludes that it's narcissism. The quote below illustrates this:

> Narcissism in relation to my features. I like my features. I'm a person who lives well with myself. If I'm alone, I'll be fine. I don't need other people to be well. For example, the activities I enjoy, I do on my own: birding, fishing [...]. I think that's to pass on my characteristics. (Milton)

I try to give degrees of importance to each of the reasons presented. Initially, Milton places the aspect of narcissism on the first level. Some time later, he places the three motives in the same order of value: perpetuation of the species/self, the desire to have many children and narcissism. The others would have the same weight (having a semen bank available for a wife's supposed need and Christian formation).

With regard to narcissism, the subject says that he appreciates his way of being, his character, his transparency and his physical appearance. According to him: "I like my manner, my character, I tend not to have any deviations in my behaviour, I try to be correct in various ways, even unlike my parents. For example, if my mum gets a fine and can 'break' it, she'll 'break' it. Not me. I go and pay it.

Regarding the character of most people, I think that many people criticise Congress, but they all act just as wrongly as the government. They criticise politicians, but if they were them they would do the same thing. He, on the other hand, is very transparent, makes it clear what he thinks and thinks that these characteristics are a great virtue.

Regarding her physical appearance, Milton thinks she's pretty. He likes her face and not so much her body. On the whole, he doesn't like the colour of her eyeballs, which have red lines, or her toes. She takes advantage of this moment when she speaks candidly about her self-impressions to once again criticise other people's behaviour. The quote below illustrates this:

> Regarding my physical appearance, I think it's beautiful. Most people say 'normal'. People generally use modesty, euphemisms. If you're going to swear at someone, you say: 'with all due respect..... '. I don't use euphemisms, because I want the person to understand what I'm saying. I speak incisively, I get straight to the point, I don't beat around the bush." (Milton)

Regarding his imperfections, in terms of personality, he sees few "defects" in himself. He says he's been through phases when he was self-interested, when he only sought people out when he needed something. At the time, his mother warned him about having the same trait as his father. Another aspect he needs to improve is the fact that he is very direct with people. However, this characteristic doesn't bother him, it bothers the other person. According to Milton: "If I have to speak, I speak and that's that, I don't keep it to myself. I get home and go to sleep.

His father seems to have more limitations than his mother. Milton says that at one point his father didn't want to pay child support. He criticised him harshly and directly: "When it came to making children, you and my mother had a lot of fun, didn't you? She liked it, you liked it, and we were born. I thank you for giving me life, I really do, but now you have to pay the alimony! Then pay it and don't complain!

I propose that we return to the main issue: the motivation for semen donation, reviewing all the steps taken. He follows and agrees with everything that has been said so far. I ask him if, as a semen donor, he expects any kind of return. He immediately replies: "No, neither affective nor financial. I'm just curious to meet the child in the future, if that's possible."

Next, I'll explain the impression their words made on me. It seemed to me that life had a positive meaning for the interviewee. He thanks his parents for the life he has been given. At this point he says: "Life is everything!". He falls silent and a great emotion emerges. I continue my reflections. In the same way that his parents gave him life, as a donor, he makes it possible for children to come into the world; he gives them existence. I ask him if he sees any meaning in this "equation". In tears, he says: "It never has, but if you say it, it could be thanks for me coming to life, but I've only just thought about it, it never came to mind. Just gratitude, and enjoying life and thinking that God is much bigger than me, that he gave me everything and never lacked anything for me. That's it". I questioned the meaning of the "everything" he had received from God. He continues: "Everything is my family, love, health, I have the financial means to live well, without going through any hardship as I know many do. Life is enough for me. I don't need anything else. In fact, at the moment, Milton feels he is missing a son.

Putting the *jigsaw* together

The data collected indicated that the interviewee decided to donate semen to a specialised bank on an impulse, or driven by emotion, being oblivious to what the act represented. According to his statement: "It just made me want to be a donor, so I typed it into Goog/and..."

As we delved deeper into his career as a semen donor, getting to know each other and becoming like-minded people, other motivations emerged and intensified.

From the initial desire to have many children, exactly five, similar to the group he was part of in the past, came the desire to relive the happy childhood he spent in an extended family of mum, sister, cousins, uncles and grandmother, where unity and love reigned. On the other hand, his descendants would fulfil several other wishes: for his continuity, for the perpetuation of humanity, and for the perpetuation of himself. To continue and multiply would be, at the same time, to pass on his characteristics, perpetuating and spreading the gift of being who he is: a good, honest, truthful, generous, affectionate, kind man who also has physical beauty, which Milton calls "narcissism". The way the subject calls himself is more about expressing a "liking of oneself" than a "liking of oneself only".

Providing semen to a bank is an act of generosity, even if the interviewee didn't want to admit it. Although he was also motivated by concern for his wife's possible future needs, Milton could have hired the service of cryopreserving his reproductive cells in the same place and for the same purpose. However, being on the company's register of anonymous donors helps it with the "raw material" for its commercial activity, and helps those women who turn to the bank with the aim of becoming pregnant.

The Christian upbringing he received from his family of origin introduced him to a creator God. Creator of everything around him, including his life and his destiny. This God gave him everything and never let him lack anything, proving to be a generous God. Even today, he feels he has "everything" and lacks nothing. Everything means: family, love, health, work, movable and immovable property, and excellent financial conditions. Yet through this God and before him, who is much greater than himself, Milton is transformed into a small, humble person, capable of bowing down to another.

We can conclude that liking life, understanding it as something positive and great, as "everything", from which the interviewee has received so many graces, so many gifts, has made him realise that he owes life thanks for having had the opportunity to experience it and to have had so much. So Milton must give back to life, for the marvellous life he has, for the marvellous man he is, giving others the opportunity to have the same experience, and endowing them with his positive predicaments.

In this sense, donating semen to unknown people for free is a way of thanking life for the gifts you have received: for everything you have had and for the good and beautiful person you are. At the same time as your reproductive cells will help infertile people have babies, they will be, albeit anonymously, your biological children (the one you still feel is missing).

He wants these children. He gives them the gift of life, the beautiful opportunity to live. On the other hand, Milton wishes to pass on to these beings his own characteristics: goodness and beauty. They fulfil his desire to have many children so that he can have continuity and immortality, so that he can relive his happy childhood with a large family. Because they are descended from different women, they will realise his desire to have children of different ethnicities, at the same time as the genitor mixes with these different "races".

Milton doesn't expect a return for the donation he made to the bank, but he would like to meet his descendants, which makes me wonder if, on a fantasy level, he wouldn't like to bring his many children together for a weekend at the children's grandmother's house, for moments of bonding and love.

The digitally recorded interview lasted one hour and forty minutes. However, we formed such an intense alliance that the impression I had was that he didn't want to let me go, but rather seemed to want to take me into his world. After the recorder was switched off, we became even more comfortable and continued the conversation. Milton asked a lot of questions about the research I was coordinating, about what he was discovering about the subject, about the progress of the search for the other subjects. For his part, he talked about his professional life, the position he holds and where he wants to go in terms of his career, starting with public examinations. He also talked about his marriage, his plans to move to a smaller, quieter city to have a better quality of life, which in turn are also my plans, and so we continued. We exchanged many affinities: the way we relate to the figure of the child, existence, sincerity... Finally, when we realised it, another two and a half hours had passed. It was almost fourteen o'clock and we'd been there since nine. It was then that Milton invited me to join him and his wife for lunch at his mum's house. I felt flattered. Unfortunately, I had to prepare for the next interview. Very touched, we said goodbye with a kiss and a big hug. Since then, whenever I remember him, his image, his watery eyes when he spoke of his existence, I feel emotion and joy at having "met" him, Milton.

The material obtained from the interview reveals that the act of donating semen to a specialised bank is part of a gift. There is a gift in the love of life, in the need to be grateful for the opportunity received, in the emotion that emerged from realising this fact, in the desire to generate lives, in the concern for his wife, for his right to motherhood, for the same concern for strangers, for helping the semen bank by providing his reproductive cells, for his relationship with divinity, for the uprightness of his character and attitudes, for the will to spread and multiply, for the love of family.

On the other hand, the difficulty that the interviewee expressed in assuming such gifts, seeking to show interest in his own person and his own universe, and denying obvious acts of giving, seem to reveal a broader issue, linked to the social construction of masculinity in Western societies, which is often related to selfishness, machismo, physical strength, virility, eroticism, and little associated with delicacy, sensitivity, kindness, generosity, altruism, selflessness, characteristics which are commonly linked to the female sex/gender.

Second meeting: **Tomaz Lins**

From our first contact, the impression I got from Tomaz was one of promptness. We met in the early evening of a Saturday, in the café of the *Livraria Cultura in the Conjunto Nacional,* the same place where I had interviewed Milton. As we only knew each other by phone, we provided information about our outfits. I wore a green dress; he wore jeans and a white T-shirt. I was at the venue by eighteen o'clock. It was an area with several tables and chairs in the centre and armchairs at the back. I was waiting in one of them, facing the entrance. It was a few minutes after the agreed time. Whenever a man arrived unaccompanied and wearing clothes like those described by Tomaz, I approached him. This happened several times, not least because "jeans and a white T-shirt" is quite common. I decided to call him without success: the answering machine came on, where I left a message.

A little more time passed and I began to notice a certain anxiety in myself as a result of the feeling that he wasn't going to turn up. I was fully aware that this feeling was a reflection of the apprehension that had accompanied me throughout my doctorate and intensified at the stage of recruiting subjects for the research.

It was nineteen o'clock. An uneasy feeling prompted me to leave the café, as it was extremely noisy and had become absolutely unfeasible for the interview. I walked from one side to the other, down a corridor that led to the entrance of the bookshop. In the *foyer* of the building I saw a very tall young man, who seemed to be over one metre and ninety centimetres tall. He was slim, light brown, had dark, well-cut hair and was wearing very modern clothes and earrings in one ear. We looked at each other and recognised each other immediately. I said: "Tomaz?". He replied: "Yes, Ana Paula. It took me a while, didn't it? But didn't I say I was coming?". I was so happy that my anxiety vanished right then and there. I proposed that we go to the terrace, where there were gardens, benches and, above all, silence. He agreed, saying he knew the place because he often went there to date. We climbed up several ramps while chatting happily. We reached the terrace level and sat down on a secluded bench. After sorting out the consent form, we began the interview.

Tomaz Lins is thirty-one years old, single, has no children, is starting a degree in accountancy and works as a school driver, responsible for transporting pupils from a school in the south of São Paulo, living in the Jardim Paulista neighbourhood. His monthly income is over R$4,000.00 (four thousand reais). He says he is an evangelical, classifies himself racially as white, and has been a semen donor for six months.

The decision to donate gametes was made for reasons that were not clear to the subject. As we went along in the interview, some assumptions were made, but these were not exchanged with Tomaz because I didn't perceive/identify any willingness on his part to do so. According to the interviewee's account:

> [...] it was something that struck me, something like that... I don't remember, I don't remember, but I think it was like this, suddenly I said: 'Let me go and look'! But it happened very quickly. When I had the intention, I went onto *Google,* searched, found it, bookmarked it. It was like that. I don't know, it gave me a strange feeling, a certain urgency, you know? How can I explain it? I felt, as if it had hit me that someone was in urgent need, so I went there. I only didn't go before because I had to stay abstinent for three or four days, otherwise I would have gone the same day. (Tomaz)

I presented the same question in different ways in order to try to "track" his sense of urgency associated with the need to supply sperm to a semen bank and, from this, the subject mentioned various hypothetical situations, but doubt was always present at the conclusion of each reasoning.

Firstly, it should be noted that, throughout our contact, Tomaz expressed his constant interest in helping people, a characteristic that was confirmed by the fact that he agreed to take part in this research.

After revealing his status as a semen donor to his mother and some friends, he received various criticisms and accusations, which he dismissed on the basis of the altruistic attitude involved in the practice. According to his speech: "Then I said so.... I think I.... at this point I'm calm, because I know I've made a family happy".

Secondly, Tomaz linked the issue to a sister's health problem and then denied it, as shown below:

> Look, maybe... it's coming to mind now... I have a sister who... she had a tubal infection, and she only had a ten per cent chance of getting pregnant naturally. That may have been what motivated me, but I don't remember if it weighed much. She's already pregnant, she's five or six weeks along, but I don't think that was it. (Tomaz)

Another possible justification for the interviewee's unwillingness to donate semen also seems to have something to do with his discouragement of marriage and, above all, fatherhood. His conviction would be linked to two issues. The first relates to a negative view of the world in which he lives. As such, Tomaz doesn't want to raise a child in a truly chaotic world. Chaos would be the result of the difficulties observed on the planet, relating to pollution, violence, mismanagement in relation to the direction of children's education and their behaviour. However, it's interesting to note that immediately afterwards, the speaker reveals a certain inconsistency and inconstancy in relation to his previous speech. The quote below illustrates this:

> Firstly, I never want to have children; I don't even want to get married [...] Look, I think the world is so difficult: violence, pollution... I work with children, I see... how children act, how education is today. It may happen, I may have a child at some point, but it's not in my plans. (Tomaz)

The other factor discouraging fatherhood reported by Tomaz is his financial problems, despite having a good monthly income, which could be due to a certain personal inability to deal with the issue. According to Tomaz: "Because I personally can't afford to have a child, I have a good income, but I spend a lot... and I have 'n' financial problems".

At one point, the interviewee asked a friend about his attitude towards donating semen, which seemed to have had some effect on him: "Ô'mêu', but don't you feel a bit remorseful knowing that suddenly, in ten years' time, you'll know that there's a child aged eight, nine, ten who has your blood and you don't know where it is?".

Trying to think about the question posed by his friend, Tomaz reveals a curious fact, based on the reasons that led him to donate sperm. He thinks of the group that undergoes treatments involving reproductive technologies as having high purchasing power, as well as financial stability, which would represent a motivating factor for him to donate semen. As Tomaz believes he is incapable of raising children, both emotionally and financially, the donation would take on the character of an exchange, in the sense that one party provides the genetic material necessary for the infertile to reproduce and the other provides the financial resources and care for the offspring. The quote below makes this clear:

> [...] to have an insemination, not just anyone can do it. You have to be in a financially secure position to have treatment, to pay for it, because it's not cheap. So I know that I didn't put my child there... it's... in the care of just anyone. The person has the means, went there, paid for it, did it and is there looking after a little seed of mine." (Tomaz)

Until the end of the interview, Tomaz didn't seem to be able to "translate" what would have led him to instantly decide to donate gametes, or even the reason for the urgency. To my question, he replied: "I don't know. I think I must have read something on the internet, from somewhere in need. It just struck me, something like that. Suddenly I said: 'Let me go and look'.

Our "meeting" revealed that Tomaz is not yet fully aware of what moved him to donate sperm to a semen bank. His personality seemed to be characterised by impulse, as he mentioned this aspect at various times: "I'm a bit like that, I feel like doing it, I go and do it!". However, the data collected provided clues that we can analyse in search of meaning.

In my opinion, Tomaz's motivation for donating semen seems to be the result of a characteristic of acting on impulse associated with various interests: the desire to act altruistically; the desire to reproduce; and the need to transfer the care of offspring to the recipients, which would relieve him of the responsibilities inherent in raising a child, which imply, at the very least, presence and financial investment.

The fact that he provides his reproductive cells, through the semen bank, to subjects who will undergo heterologous artificial insemination, would represent the realisation of the donor's interests, because through the recipient individuals, Tomaz will be able to practise altruism, helping an infertile subject to give birth, while also reproducing himself. On the other hand, the donor transfers the responsibilities required by paternity to the recipient, which is in the interests of both parties.

Third meeting: **Edu José**

Edu proved to be a very approachable guy from the very beginning of our contact in July 2009. Every time I sent him an *email,* it was answered immediately and objectively.

The scheduled date for our interview was November, but it was brought forward to October due to a national holiday that lasted from Saturday to Tuesday. During that period Edu came to Rio de Janeiro on a tourist trip.

The subject had sent *an email* informing me of his trip and of the possibility of giving me the interview already planned here, in the city where I live, which would resolve the issue of physical space, mentioned earlier. The message provided all the information about his whereabouts. He would be staying in a neighbourhood close to my home, where I would receive him. The interview was scheduled for early Sunday evening.

I spent a long time setting up the place where the interview would take place: the living room, so that the environment would inspire as much neutrality as possible. So I removed photos, knick-knacks and other personal objects, leaving only the furniture: a sofa, a hermetically sealed bookcase and a table with two chairs. The doors to all the other rooms were closed. *Food and drink* were placed on the table.

I arranged to pick him up from where he was staying. On the appointed date, time and place, I phoned him and told him I was waiting for him in front of the building. A few minutes later, two boys turned up. It was Edu with a friend, Lúcio, to whom I was introduced. I greeted him nicely and he went back inside the building. He seemed to have come down to see me, which was later confirmed by the interviewee. He left and Edu and I headed for my car.

We chatted a lot on the quick journey to the interview venue. When we arrived, Edu chose to stay at the table. I gave him two copies of the consent form, which he signed and distributed to the parties. We then began recording.

Edu José is twenty-eight years old, has a degree in chemical engineering, works as a consulting engineer for a company located in the interior of São Paulo, and lives in the same city: Praia Grande. He is single, has no children and his monthly income is around R$4,000.00 (four thousand reais). He has no religious beliefs and doesn't even believe in a God. He classifies himself as white and has been donating semen at the same bank for seven years.

I conducted the interview in the same way as the others. I started by asking for their personal details and went on to the topics in the script. We continued in this order for a while, until Edu asked if he could talk about what led him to donate semen. I readily agreed and he began, making it clear that he felt a certain urgency to talk about the subject.

The interviewee began with an account of an existential conflict that took place during his childhood. When he was around four years old, Edu remembers being aware of his life, his individuality and his death, which would have happened at the time of his grandmother's death. See the quote below:

> Well, since I was four years old, five years old, five, six years old, it's... I realised that I was alive. I realised that I was alive, that I was me, that my father was my father, and that I was going to die one day. That's when I got a bit upset, that I was going to die. I realised that I was alive, that there was a life.... It was more or less when my grandmother died that I realised it was going to happen to me too. Then I started asking myself, right? What that was like. If there was life after death, if you had to have a religion, if you had to believe in the Bible to be able to go to heaven, if there was paradise, if lions really lived with zebras in paradise, things like that. (Edu)

The quote above shows how much Edu's process of becoming aware of the life/death cycle generated obscure feelings of fear, insecurity, anxiety and impotence, among others. In an attempt to resolve this situation of anguish, the boy sought support in the religious beliefs of the people he lived with, whose beliefs were out of sync within his family, reinforcing the state of confusion identified in the child. The maid, an evangelical, said that hell was the right place for those who didn't attend her church. His grandmother told him that he had to become a Catholic to gain salvation. His mother was a spiritualist, who instructed him to believe in spirits as proof of the existence of life after death. His father, an atheist, said that he didn't need to believe in anything and that he would still go to heaven. At that point, all Edu had to do was accept all the religious versions provided.

Time passed and Edu's conflicts subsided. However, during his teenage years, the theme of the life/death cycle came up again. At this point, he turned to his father for explanations. Roberto (the father) spoke of the existence of various religions and belief in them as a matter of choice. His view of the subject was based on materialistic ideas, from which faith made no sense, since neither the veracity of faith nor the existence of God was scientifically proven.

It's worth pointing out that Edu's father had also experienced a drama related to religion during his childhood and adolescence. Roberto lived with his family in a town in the interior of Santa Catarina, and there the figure of the priest had the power of governance. Roberto's father, Edu's grandfather, used to have intense and constant conflicts with the priest, which led to terrible arguments between the two parties. Ever since he was a boy, Roberto used to witness the countless and torrential disagreements between his father and the priest, which left him with an unending feeling of hurt. As a result, the family ended up moving to another city, São Paulo, where the church had a lower *status than in* their home town.

Edu explains that this experience caused his father such deep hurt that the feeling remains with him to this day.

At the time of defining his professional life, when the same conflicts were still present and intense, Edu decided to study biology in order to understand the mechanisms of the human body. The quote elucidates the above:

> I was left wondering if I believed or not. I was very unsure at the time and then I decided to study biology to learn a bit more about how the human body worked, what cells were like, cell reproduction, mitosis, meiosis, how people grew, everything, right? (Edu)

As he didn't pass the first entrance exam for biology, he went on to study chemical engineering at the second, from which he was selected for a scientific initiation in biology, and then devoted himself to research into animal genetics. In his studies of DNA, Edu learnt about cellular modification, the shortening of telomeres[28] , the degradation of chromosomes, the gradual loss of genetic memory, the appearance of diseases, the ageing of the skin and the death of the organism. It's interesting to note that, when describing the process of cellular modification, Edu replaces the end of the organism with the expression "everything", which seems to reflect the difficulty in

[28] Telomeres are structures made up of repetitive rows of proteins and non-coding DNA located at the ends of chromosomes. Their main function is to maintain the structural stability of the chromosome (CAMPBELL, 2001).

dealing with the subject of "death" in question. The following quote illustrates this:

> [...] then I started to learn that in cellular modification there are telomeres, and telomeres get shorter as time goes by. This ends up degrading the chromosomes and you end up losing genetic memory. This creates various diseases and even skin degradation, and then the... everything [...]. (Edu)

Edu then reports on another process relating to the degradation of the organism, now related to oxygen: in the reactions that lead to the production of energy by the mitochondria[29] , the O2 molecule (oxygen + oxygen) is broken into two parts, releasing highly reactive substances called free radicals. When these radicals react with the constituents of the mitochondria, they cause damage to its structures and a reduction in its ability to produce energy, resulting in cellular ageing, also known as oxidation. Nowadays, defence mechanisms against the harmful action of these free radicals are favoured, such as the use of *vitamin C,* for example.

According to the interviewee, there is an American movement that emphasises abstinence from physical exercise and radical dietary restrictions, turning its followers into walking skeletons as a way of prolonging life.

Edu judges this way of living as "dumb", due to its extreme restrictions. However, the interviewee would have found his own way of "circumventing" death, in the midst of scientific explanations, through reproduction. According to his account:

> [...] And *then,* in all this searching, I realised that... how could I circumvent death, since it's inevitable, the way to circumvent death is to have children, right? So, what I began to realise is that we're here, our ancestors, they had children and passed their material on, and I began to realise that we're here just for that, to have children and that's it. What we do extra is overtime, you know? All the progress we've made to date, computers, television, videos, all the things that revolve around them, that's the extra hour you're putting in, right? Now, those who really had to do it were born, reproduced and died. So reproducing is the main mission in life, you know?

Based on the above, I asked him about his opinion of people who live and don't procreate, to which Edu replied: "They haven't fulfilled their mission here on Earth."

The terms of his statement make it clear that the way the interviewee found to "circumvent" death is based on keeping his genetic material in circulation, in reproduction, in the production of children. We'll see that the factor that motivated Edu to donate semen refers to the generation of descendants who, in turn, will guarantee the continuity of the genitor, at a certain level. According to his account: "[...] That's what I think and as I still didn't have a girlfriend, I didn't realise what the future would be , so I

[29] Mitochondria are microscopic organelles found in all the body's cells and are responsible for energy production (CAMPBELL, 2001).

started donating, because at least there's a chance of me having a child, you know?".

Edu's explanations of his motivation for donating semen, which are linked to his life story, remained based on science and technology, with the human body as the main focus. As such, it was to be expected that he would attribute all aspects of transmission through procreation to genetics. It's common to see materialistic discourses from individuals whose worldview is based on materialism.

According to Edu, this kind of idea about the constitution of physical and subjective aspects as being genetic is common in biology circles, with which he partially agrees. For him, a child's upbringing is a determining factor in the formation of their character and personality. According to his account,

> Biologists have a lot of faith in this, in the idea that everything is genetic, right? I think that some aspects are true, but nobody can tell you that raising a child or not raising a child is going to change anything, you know? When you raise a child, you're going to change something, there's no way. I think that if I raise my child, it's going to be very different than if someone else raises it.

Taking Edu's testimony as a basis, and seeking to understand the factors related to his desire to donate sperm to a semen bank, we can conclude that he sees the production of children as a "life mission"; a resource that aims to alleviate (but not resolve) his conflicts resulting from the reality of the finitude of human life, or death in the future as a fait accompli, conflicts that were triggered in his first years of life. Donating gametes to be used by individuals who wish to procreate and are unable to do so naturally represents a guarantee of continuity for the deponent, albeit genetically, since their participation in the arrangement is anonymous.

In my opinion, the conflicts that began in childhood have accompanied Edu throughout his life.

life and are still present today. This is evident in the following story:

> [...] but I think that life is something we have, I think we have to preserve it, it's what we have and we don't know... what I've really come to realise is that we don't know if there is life after death, if there is paradise, if we're really going to heaven or hell. That's the conclusion I've drawn from all this since I was four years old. So, just in case, let's do what we have to do [reproduce]. (Edu)

In addition, when he contacted me after the interview had finished, Edu still tried to ask me about my religious beliefs and my ideas on the question of life and death, showing that the issue that originated many years ago is still central to his life.

Finally, it's worth pointing out that, as with the first subject, the data collected showed that Edu José also has a certain difficulty in self-attributing attitudes and intentions linked to the gift sphere.

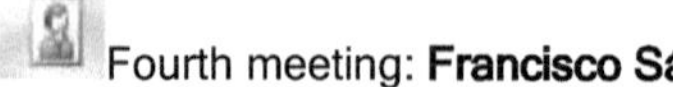

Fourth meeting: **Francisco Sá**

Contact with Francisco began in July 2009, when he sent me an *email* offering to take part in the research. However, it was difficult to schedule an appointment, as he was always unable to turn up.

As I said earlier, travelling to São Paulo was not an easy or routine task, and it meant certain personal and financial inconveniences. On the first date I suggested, the impossibilities were so great and extended to every hour of every day, that I even proposed over the phone that we have dinner together, when we would then do the interview. At some point, that man would have to stop working to eat, I thought. He found it funny and said: "It doesn't have to be like that either. We can have dinner, that's fine, but... I'll make an appointment, I'll make an appointment!".

The planned date was cancelled due to a personal health problem. However, the subsequent dialogues took on a different character. The frequent difficulties were replaced by availability. So we scheduled our meeting for fourteen o'clock on a Friday, shortly after my arrival in the city.

As there were to be interviews with three subjects over two days (Friday and Saturday), I had to stay in a hotel, where the agents were also welcomed. As soon as I settled into the room, I hid personal items such as my suitcase, handbag, toiletries, food, as well as my bed linen and bath towels. My aim was to leave the room relatively neutral. In the room, I allocated an anteroom consisting of a table and two chairs as the interview location.

A few minutes after the scheduled time, reception announced Francisco's arrival. I stood at the door to wait for him, while I realised the emotion that always inhabited me at moments like that: yet another subject was arriving to enrich the research I was coordinating.

I saw a very different man to the one I had imagined, because Francisco is a *jiu-jitsu* fighter and I had imagined him to be long. He is a very strong man, weighing over a hundred kilograms and of medium height, probably around one metre and seventy centimetres tall. The agent is twenty-six years old, married, has no children, has only studied advertising and publicity for two years, and currently works as a secretary for a doctor who is dedicated to academic research and teaching. As well as this occupation,

Francisco teaches *jiu-jitsu to* children and young people, which he sees as his true vocation and with which he intends to work exclusively in the future.

Francisco Sá is responsible for the family's expenses, since his wife doesn't work, and his monthly income amounts to an average of R$2,500.00 (two thousand five hundred reais). He lives in the Butantã neighbourhood of São Paulo, classifies himself racially as brown/light brown and calls himself an atheist. He has been a semen donor for eleven months.

We took the consent form as usual and then switched on the tape recorder. The first few minutes of the interview were marred by two unforeseen events. Firstly, I noticed that the recorder wasn't working normally and seemed to be paused. The batteries were replaced with new ones, the "REC" button was pressed again and the device was still switched off. Francisco, who calls himself an *expert* in technological matters, fiddled with the recorder's mechanisms and got it to work.

Once the problem had been solved, we restarted the interview. After two and a half minutes, the interviewee's mobile rang and I encouraged him to answer. His wife was on the other end of the line and said that the electricity at the couple's home would be cut off at any moment, according to a notice from the São Paulo electricity company, and that he should sort it out. Given the seriousness of the situation, I suggested that we move our interview to a later date, but Francisco opted to continue.

The man reports that he decided to donate sperm after reading an advert in a newspaper with a wide circulation in his city, in which a semen bank was asking for men with a certain profile to do so, with the aim of providing help to infertile people who want to procreate through reproductive technologies.

Two factors moved Francisco to comply with the terms of the advert published by the semen bank. The first is related to his enormous desire to have a child. This (the child) occupies one of the highest levels in the life of the interviewee, in terms of importance, surpassed only by achieving financial stability. And even the goal of rising economically is closely linked to the future he wants to offer his offspring. According to his account:

> In terms of importance in my life, the child is fundamental. For me, it's financial stability and the second is having a child. Because... you're going to have a child and not worry about stabilising yourself? Then you're going to raise your child by leaps and bounds. You'll lack things, you won't be able to give them a good education, they'll suffer in the future, underemployed. So it's stabilising and having a child. That's it for me (Francisco)

Francisco's second motivating factor towards the practice of semen donation was the altruistic feeling that emerged when he thought of an individual who wanted to have a baby as much as he did and, due to health problems, was unable to reproduce. The following quote illustrates this:

> The main motivating factor for donating semen, I think, was to help my neighbour. I think it's cool. I'm dying to be a father. Soon, after two years of marriage, I want to be a father e.... imagine a guy who can't, has a problem .... So I think it's helping, I think it's perfect. If the guy is going to stay
> happy having a child, like that, okay! That's what I donated it for. (Francisco)

Francisco was very objective when giving his opinions. His answers were often monosyllabic. He understands life from a materialistic point of view, according to which "what I haven't seen, I don't believe in", or "it's dead, it's over, and I've never stopped to try and look into it". Due to the concreteness of life, according to the interviewee, his son would occupy a place of importance because he represents the continuity of his existence.

I made a few attempts to delve deeper into his ideas, opinions and, above all, the question of his desire to donate semen, but he was adamant about going beyond what we had said. I asked him if the unforeseen problem with the light in his house had interfered with the interview. He replied: "No, no. I'm like that, very objective. Yes, yes. No, it's not.

After twenty-one minutes, our meeting ended as follows:

> Ana Paula: Did this research make you think of anything?
> Francisco: No, no. It hasn't changed at all.
> Ana Paula: Do you want to finish with any comments?
> Francisco: That's it!

Fifth meeting: **Ivan Pessoa**

Ivan Pessoa was the person I communicated with most during the period when the interview appointment was on hold. He never replied to my *emails*, but he used to talk for a long time on the phone. In our contacts, Ivan was always very helpful, making himself available for whatever was needed for the research. The typical phrase he used was: "Ana, I'm here. You just have to define where and when, and I'll go!".

We scheduled our interview for early Friday evening, at 8pm, when the subject was announced from reception. Within a few minutes I heard knocks on the door, it opened, and both of us were perplexed in disguise. His image was quite different from the one built up in my imagination. The reverse was probably true. We greeted each other and proceeded with the usual consent form. Then we began the interview.

Ivan is forty-seven years old, divorced, has a degree in mechanical engineering, continues his father's work by coordinating a company that produces industrial parts, lives alone in the São Paulo neighbourhood of Alto da Lapa, and has a monthly income of R$2,300.00 (two thousand three hundred reais) on average. He has been a semen donor for four years and racially classifies himself as white.

Of all the agents, Ivan was the oldest donor, as well as the most "open-minded", benevolent and accepting of others. He is characterised as a very talkative individual. In his speech, one thought always leads to many others. So I had to direct the interview a lot so that we didn't lose focus.

As soon as the recorder was switched on, the subject started asking questions about the field of semen donation, demonstrating that he had very little knowledge of the subject. Spontaneously, he began to talk about the factors that motivated him to donate semen: the fact that he was a regular blood donor, and the fact that he liked helping people, led him to look for other ways of donating human material. When he turned to the *Google* search engine, *he* got results for bone marrow donation and semen donation. He was immediately interested in the second option.

Ivan not only donates blood and semen, but also takes part in various surveys: opinion polls, pharmaceutical industry surveys and many others. His philosophy of life translates into altruistic attitudes. He believes that human existence itself is justified by helping others on a collective level. However, in his opinion, human beings are "very stupid" because they are extremely individualistic. In his opinion, he "doesn't have his feet on the ground much" and so he likes to help his neighbour, even if that neighbour is a mere stranger, which is confirmed in the quote below:

> I think, well... Human beings have to help each other, right? I think that's what we're here for. Wars, everything, everything, everything happens here on Earth, with us, here, because of that, right? Because nobody helps each other. No-one! I don't know... Human beings are very stupid, very, very stupid. But I'm not, you know, Ana? I am, I am I don't really have my feet on the ground. I'm a bit... I don't know, of suddenly you understand... I really go for the human side of things. (Ivan)

The interviewee explains that he was motivated to donate his reproductive cells to a semen bank because he wanted to help people who couldn't have a baby naturally. There is another factor: Ivan is the father of three children. The eldest is twenty years old and the youngest is six. There is another girl, who is now eighteen. He says that his children have always been a source of great personal fulfilment. Based on his own feelings about fatherhood, he says that he wants the infertile individual to be able to feel what he himself felt when he saw his firstborn for the first time, and to be able to experience the pleasures that fatherhood offers: bearing a child, seeing it born and grow, and becoming a great companion. The following quote illustrates the point:

> So I've already told you that, because I want to see... I don't want to see it, I don't see it, but in reality, I'd like someone to have the same feeling I had when I saw my son in the maternity ward. The paediatrician opened the little window and showed me my son. [...] No, but that's it. I want, I'd really like, someone else, other people, whether they're men or women, to have the same feeling I had, the pleasure I had in having a child, bearing a child, you know? And then, in reality, I know that there are people who have difficulties, don't get pregnant, try, I don't know what and so on. So I think, well, why not? I won't know who it is. I don't need to. Knowing that I collaborated is fine!" (Ivan)

Ivan sees semen donation as a praiseworthy act, not because he is one of the representatives of the class, but solely and exclusively because it helps someone else realise a dream, because it eases the feelings of sadness of someone who is infertile, because it can be a vehicle for the birth of a new life, which turns the act into something noble.

In the course of the interview, when we talked about the topic of "religion", a new aspect of the desire to donate semen emerged. Ivan is not an adherent of any religion, brotherhood or sect, he just believes in God, in a creator God.

Throughout his life, he tried to get closer to various types of religion or spiritualism. Ivan studied for many years at a priest's school, as a boarder, dedicated himself to Catholicism, got to know Spiritism, attended the *Seicho-No-ie*, the Brazilian Congregation, the Christian Communication in Brazil, the Evangelical Church, among others, but he didn't feel in tune with any religious practice. According to the interviewee, everyone is looking for a God, and everyone believes in God. For him, God is enough, because he is the creator of the world and of human beings.

As Ivan spoke about God, the look on his face changed and a strong emotion became visible. An intense feeling reverberated in me too. I asked him if he kept in touch with this God, the one we were talking about. The interviewee said that not only does he keep in touch with God, but he has been certain of his existence through several of his experiences, which brought out the latent emotion. Ivan says the following about his connection with God:

> With God? Absolutely! Not just contact, but I have proof that he exists through various things that have happened to me, and for me, it was he who did it. He kept me. I've been to.... When I had the accident, I had to die... I don't know, various things. It was he who took away my father's pain, three days before he died... I think so. I'm sure of it. Not only do I think it, I'm sure of it. (Ivan)

I think Ivan Pessoa's strong connection with the creator God makes him sensitive to the suffering of others. His closeness to this God makes him benevolent. Being good to others brings him self-contentment. In essence, his philosophy of life, centred on altruistic attitudes, reflects his desire to serve God by giving of himself to those in need, and this giving of himself returns to the point of origin in the form of personal well-being.

He points out that the way of being he cultivates doesn't serve to maximise him in the eyes of his peers. He only does what he thinks is right. In his words:

> And that's it, I don't know. I'm no more than anyone else because I believe in God, because I'm a semen donor. I feel nothing, nothing, nothing, nothing more than anyone else, than a human being, but whatever I can do, I do for others, to feel good, to serve God. If I think it's valid, I do it." (Ivan)

We ended our meeting under the impact of emotion. Him, for being who he is. Me, for having surrendered to his sensitivity.

We talked for a while and would have stayed longer if Ivan hadn't had to go and help his mum, who had phoned him during the interview. She was lonely. She had only been a widow for a few days. We said goodbye, I took him to the door and gave him a hug, saying: "I really enjoyed meeting you". He shyly replied: "I really enjoyed meeting you too. And if there's anything you need, just give me a call".

 Sixth meeting: **Luiz Cláudio**

Luiz Cláudio volunteered to take part in the field study stage, giving his testimony, but scheduling the interview was an arduous task. His justifications were based on his long periods of dedication to work, then due to his holidays abroad. But finally, the meeting took place at the beginning of my last day in São Paulo.

At eight o'clock in the morning, the hotel reception called my room to inform me of the arrival of Luiz Cláudio, whom I had invited to breakfast. As he was coming from a distant neighbourhood and had only made that time available for the interview, I thought it would be kind of me to offer him breakfast. I went downstairs straight away, we greeted each other happily as we were getting to know each other face-to-face, and headed for the lounge, where we chatted a lot about his life (work, family, professionalisation, expectations for the future), as well as about the ongoing research and the day-to-day life of a PhD student. There was a relaxed atmosphere between us. We then went to the interview location and started recording.

Luiz Cláudio is thirty-six years old, single and lives with his family: father, mother and three sisters in the Interlagos neighbourhood of São Paulo. He graduated in business administration and holds the same position where he works. His personal income varies around R$2,300.00 (two thousand three hundred reais), while the family income is around R$7,000.00 (seven thousand reais). He has no children, calls himself an "eclectic Catholic" and, when asked to classify himself racially, he was embarrassed by the fact that his ancestry is ethnically varied. At first, Luiz said he didn't know what to say. Later, he said he wasn't a "legitimate black" and finalised by defining himself as "brown". He has also been a semen donor for a year.

Luiz says that he had heard about the subject of gamete donation on television and in magazines, but not much, because it is a subject that is not widely publicised. One day, a friend shared with him the drama experienced by a sister who couldn't get pregnant with her husband due to an immunological factor, i.e. there was an incompatibility between cervical mucus and sperm. As the woman wanted to have a child, the couple resorted to heterologous artificial insemination to realise their intention. Three years of attempts and a favourable outcome: the baby was born.

As he listened to the story, Luiz Cláudio formulated a thesis. As he isn't married and doesn't even have a girlfriend, the chances of him becoming a father at the moment are very remote. In this sense, the donation of semen would have an exchange function: by providing his reproductive cells to the semen bank, Luiz would be acting in favour of someone who wants to have a child and, due to infertility, is unable to do so. In return, the woman who will benefit from his gametes will be repaying him with a descendant. The quote below illustrates this:

> [...] And there's that old story... I don't know if it's a psychological thing or not, but it's like this, as I've always liked this family thing, all this stuff, and as I don't have children or anything, it goes, right? So in my heart, I imagine it like this: Oh well, there's a little son of mine out there, right? Spread out, but more in this sense, of being able to help others and, psychologically, to help my inner self too, in this sense. (Luiz Cláudio)

As soon as he could, driven by enormous curiosity, he turned to the internet to find out about the subject, found the semen bank, and in a few days came forward to donate. Today, he is living in expectation of the existence of this descendant. This became clear at the very beginning of the interview, when personal details were collected, under "child". At the time, the intention was to find out if he had a child. Luiz replied: "I don't think so!" while laughing a lot, expressing a double meaning in his speech. The possibility that he was already a father through donated semen was the biased message of his response.

Luiz Cláudio is also satisfied with his *status* as a semen donor. Partly for the other person, who has achieved a goal. Partly for himself, for having helped his fellow man. In addition, in his opinion, the practice offers gains related to the idea that his offspring will be raised by individuals from higher social strata, which will favour a higher level of education than the biological father could offer. According to his account:

> I'm happy for the others. Because I'm happy for myself, knowing that I've been able to help someone, right? Who really wants to be a mum, a dad and all that, and also for the person who really doesn't have the possibility of having a child, with their dad, with their partner and so on, so they have it some other way. Since you know, even more so since you've been through this whole process, you know that a child has gone to a family that can give, I don't know.... I know it's long-term, right? A good upbringing for your child, everything else, maybe even better than you could have given them yourself, or if you're lucky enough to get one, a father, a mother who are very good. (Luiz Cláudio)

In this sense, based on the interviewee's statement, it can be seen that Luiz Cláudio became a semen donor, motivated by an idea of an alliance between donor and recipient, which would result in an "exchange of favours". The infertile individual receives reproductive cells from the fertile one, which will fulfil the former's desire to reproduce. The latter, in return, generates the child that contains the genetic load of both parties, giving the donor the satisfaction of having the *status of* father. At the end of the investigation, Luiz presents another category of gift coming from the recipient: the latter, who, because he is a user of CRTs, would occupy the position of the wealthy in the donor's imagination, will offer the child a higher standard of living compared to the economic possibilities of the biological father.

The contact established with Luiz drew my attention to a very characteristic behaviour of the subject: that of frequently associating some kind of joke with his answers, which may be indicating the existence of a difficulty in broaching the subject, not least because, according to his testimony, the event had never been mentioned to anyone else before our "meeting".

5.4 **Discussion and analysis of the data**

The data presented below was collected because of its relevance to the contextualisation of this research.

Of the six interviews conducted, whose script consisted of sixteen topics, the item corresponding to the subject of this study was selected as a category: *the agents' motivation for donating semen.* In addition to the main category, fifteen aspects were raised. These are knowledge about the subject of the research (HTs and gamete donation); opinion about the donation of reproductive cells; approach to the practice of donation; experience with sperm donation at the semen bank; knowledge and opinion about the regulation of the practice (gratuity and anonymity); semen donation and social relations; opinion on the users of their semen (heterosexuals, homosexuals, singles and older people); the destination of donated semen (from collection to baby); representation of the child; donor and the child resulting from the donation; donor as recipient; religion; donor profile; motivation for taking part in the research; some questions about race.

These fifteen aspects were addressed in the interviews so that they could be related to the main category and serve as support in analysing the data collected.

5.4.1 Analysis of the aspects collected, related to the main category

5.4.1.1 Socio-demographic data

The six men interviewed for this research are between twenty-six and forty-seven years old, with half of them between twenty-six and twenty-eight, two others between thirty-one and thirty-six and the oldest: forty-seven.

All of the interviewees have higher education qualifications, one of whom is still at university and the other who has been enrolled on a course for two years. The professions chosen were: law, accounting, advertising, business administration and chemical and mechanical engineering. Two of them work in activities other than their professional training. The accounting student works as a school driver, responsible for transporting pupils to and from school. The other, who is not enrolled in an advertising course, works as a secretary for a medical researcher (typing up texts, preparing lectures and presentations, buying equipment and whatever else is necessary). In his spare time, he also teaches *jiu-jitsu* to children and young people, as well as taking part in heavyweight competitions.

Half the group is single, one is divorced and the remaining two have been married for two years. One of the women works and the other is a housewife. The divorced man and two of the single men live alone. The other single man lives with his father, mother and three sisters. The married men live only with their wives. Only the divorced man has children, a total of three.

Four donors live in the following neighbourhoods in the city of São Paulo: Alto da Lapa, Interlagos, Jardim Paulista and Butantã. One of them lives in Praia Grande, a municipality in São Paulo, and the other in the Higienópolis neighbourhood in São José do Rio Preto.

The group's personal income ranges from R$ 2,300.00 (two thousand three hundred reais) to R$ 4,500.00 (four thousand five hundred reais), with the amount for families varying between R$ 2,500 (two thousand five hundred reais) and R$ 7,000.00 (seven thousand reais).

As for the length of experience with the practice of semen donation, the data collected indicates variability on the subject. The shortest period of experience investigated was six months. The longest period found was seven years. As for the other interviewees, two have been registered with the bank for a year, the third has been a donor for eleven months and the last has been donating semen for four years.

In terms of "race", the collection of material was limited to the racial self-classification of the subjects, since the subject, although relevant, was not prioritised in this study. According to the results, the majority of donors classified themselves as "white". Only two called themselves "brown", "light brown", "brunette" and "non-legitimate black".

It was interesting to note that for the "non-white" interviewees, assigning themselves a "colour" or "race" proved to be a difficult task, while for the others, racial self-classification occurred almost automatically.

The results obtained in relation to the topics investigated in the fieldwork will be presented below, along with a brief discussion of some issues relating to "race" in Brazil. Subsequently, the data collected will be analysed in relation to the study category in subsection 5.4.2.

5.4.1.2 Knowledge on the topic: conceptive reproductive technologies and donation of gametes

The aim of collecting data on this subject was to investigate the level of knowledge that the interviewees have about gamete donation and the subject to which the practice belongs: conceptive reproductive technologies. The study of the subject made it possible to assess the extent to which having information on the subject would have aroused the subject's interest in semen donation, or the opposite.

According to the data collected, the six interviewees have a very superficial level of knowledge about the subject. Most of the time, they didn't even understand the question, or tried to answer it based on their experience with semen donation, or even personal speculation. For illustrative purposes, I transcribe below a fragment of the dialogue between Edu and myself:

> [What knowledge do you have about reproductive technologies and gamete donation? "I know very little. I have very little knowledge. What I do know is

> that... semen donation is used by infertile people who want to procreate. Donated semen is also used in illegal research, for cloning, embryo research, stem cells, things like that [...].

According to Francisco: "I have little knowledge. I've never read anything about it. I know that egg donation also exists, that semen donation is anonymous, and that it's to help infertile couples who can't have children, and who do artificial insemination. That's all."

Two interviewees said that the little knowledge they had was the result of their contact with the semen bank. According to Milton's statement, "the little knowledge I have came from contact with the semen bank, through the questions I asked, which were all answered, which were about anonymity, the tests required of the donor and I was told that the semen is sent to clinics". Milton also said that he had read something about the regulation of gamete donation at the bank itself, but that he couldn't remember anything about it.

Ivan and Luiz Cláudio only know what they experienced during the semen collection process, when practically nothing was questioned. The latter doesn't even know the meaning of the word "gamete".

It's worth pointing out that Ivan took advantage of the interview to ask a lot of questions about the subject, since during his contact with the semen bank he felt that the management was rather reserved when it came to passing on information on the subject. Ivan's attitude was repeated by the other agents, who ended up using the meetings to increase their level of knowledge about ART and gamete donation.

5.4.1.3 Opinion on gamete donation

The aim of this topic was to find out what these men think about gamete donation (eggs and semen). It was expected that the answers would be limited to favourable/unfavourable. However, as it was a topic and not a closed question, there was room for other comments that seemed relevant to the interviewees.

With regard to semen and egg donation, half of the group interviewed (Ivan, Tomaz and Francisco) are in favour of the practice as a TRC resource, due to the fact that it helps infertile individuals on the one hand and promotes the birth of human beings on the other.

One of the subjects has no opinion. Milton confines himself to thinking of the practice of gamete donation as "a matter of choice for each person". Edu shares this idea, as he feels personal satisfaction with the fact that his semen is stored and distributed to those who request it.

According to Luiz Cláudio, semen and egg donation should be more widely publicised in the mass media, because "the general public is either unaware of the subject or has a distorted understanding of it".

Tomaz adds that acting as a gamete donor requires a psychological balance, in order to deal with the consequences of this attitude. According to Tomaz, services aimed at assessment and psychological support should be made available to all individuals involved in heterologous reproduction: donors, recipients, children born and employees. These services should be included in all institutions specialising in the practice, such as semen banks, clinics and hospitals specialising in reproductive technologies. For the interviewee, donating semen can be seen both as an act of sanity, because it aims to help people, and as an act of insanity, because of the countless results it produces.

5.4.1.4 Getting closer to the practice of semen donation

The aim of this topic was to find out how each of the subjects came to have closer ties with semen donation.

Based on the data collected, five of the six subjects decided to donate semen for personal reasons. Only one (Francisco) approached the practice for external reasons, prompted by a newspaper advert for a semen bank, through which semen donors were solicited.

As for the other five, three of them (Milton, Tomaz and Edu) felt an internal need to donate semen, which led them to look on the internet for a place of reference, *on* the *Google* search *engine.* They found a semen bank in São Paulo that is the most representative in the country and, through its web address, they made contact, received information about the donation process, booked appointments and followed through with the procedures required by the clinic specialising in the subject, until they became part of the company's donor register.

The other two interviewees (Ivan and Luiz Cláudio), who also sought semen donation for personal reasons, did so in a different way. One of them was already a regular blood donor and felt attracted to donating another type of human material. He turned to *Google* and got results for bone marrow donation and semen donation. He immediately opted for gamete donation because it promotes human reproduction. The other subject had his curiosity aroused after hearing a story about a case of heterologous artificial insemination, which involved many difficulties but was successful. Both interviewees arrived at the semen bank through *Google* searches, where they travelled the same path as the three previous interviewees.

5.4.1.5 Regulating the practice: free of charge and anonymity

The aim of this topic was to investigate the level of knowledge that the group studied has about the standardisation of both TRCs and the rules on anonymity and gratuity. It also sought to address the subjects' opinions on the subject.

Of all the people interviewed, five (Tomaz, Edu, Ivan, Francisco and Luiz Cláudio) were unaware of the regulations that standardise gamete donation in Brazil. The other, Milton, who is a lawyer, recalled having read something about the subject when he visited the semen bank, but could no longer remember. During the investigation, the subject was given a *folder* advertising the bank, which summarised the issue. Milton read the material and then spoke up.

In his opinion, only the law can regulate a practice like gamete donation, which involves so many controversies and polemics, which are related to the rule of anonymity. For Milton, semen donation (as well as egg donation) is not something that can be done on the sly, and because the donor doesn't just donate cells, he donates everything of himself: gametes, phenotypic characteristics, subjective traits such as character, temperament, among others.

According to the interviewee, the Brazilian Constitution advocates the right of every individual to have their paternity recognised, as well as the right of all people to know their biological origins. In this sense, the anonymity rule, guided by the current CFM resolution, would be acting in the opposite direction, denying this right to people born through donated gametes, which would be unfair to them. The Constitution and the ECA (Statute of the Child and Adolescent) are instruments that can be used by this discriminated group to bring legal proceedings in which they can claim their right. Depending on the judge's understanding, the semen bank will have to provide the donors' details. The donors, in turn, will have to appear in court if they are summoned. If the semen donation is kept secret, the donor could have problems with his family, which is not the case with Milton, who chose to reveal the situation to his family.

Still according to Milton, the ideal would be to have optional anonymity, which would work as "pure" or as "conditioned". The individual who opted for "pure anonymity" would be choosing the situation we are currently experiencing: the parties would not be in contact.

However, the individual who opted for the "conditional anonymity" type would be agreeing to contact with the party receiving the semen donation.

Edu José disagrees with the anonymity rule. For his part, he would like to meet all the children born through his donated semen, and it would be in his interest to live with them. According to his statement: "Even if the director of the bank gave me a list of the people who have my children, I'd contact them one by one, and I'd make a point of hanging out with the kids and everything. I'd even like to take part [...]",

The remaining four interviewees: Ivan, Luiz Cláudio, Francisco and Tomaz agree with anonymity, albeit in different ways. The first two were open to the possibility of contacting their descendants. Tomaz, on the other hand, prefers not to meet them. Francisco doesn't have the same interest as the first two, but he would accept breaking his anonymity if it was important to the child, but only with the authorisation of the receiving parents. Still on the subject, Luiz Cláudio explains that because semen donors are undifferentiated subjects in practice and in the production of the baby, they are reduced to the condition of "breeding bulls".

All the interviewees were in favour of the donation being free of charge, and made the donation with total disinterest in any kind of return, but there were reservations. Milton was in favour of providing a stipend to those who need it, with criteria so that it doesn't become a type of indirect remuneration. This allowance would be used to cover the financial and time investments that every donor needs to make to attend the various visits required by the semen bank, where there are costs for transport, parking for those who use a car and food, as some time is spent on each visit.

Ivan has a similar opinion to Milton. According to him, the semen bank should reciprocate the donor's noble attitude, but in a symbolic way. In the same way that research institutes do, where the agent has a lot of experience as a researcher, the bank could reimburse the costs of the donors travelling and, in addition, it would be nice to be offered a snack after collecting the sperm, and/or some kind of gift that would represent a kind of thank you, such as a pen with the company logo on it, for example, with the following phrase on it: "Your attitude helped someone come into the world".

According to Ivan, another way of repaying the donor's gesture would be to offer them warmer treatment when they visit the site. At the end of the material collection, as opposed to leaving alone, there should be a company employee to say thank you and goodbye to the subject.

Edu has the same complaint as Ivan. He also says that he would like to have more privacy during his visits to the semen bank, which would be a way of encouraging the donor.

For three of the interviewees (Ivan, Edu and Milton), the free-of-charge rule may be contributing to the shortage of men wishing to donate semen.

5.4.1.6 Semen donation and social relations

The aim of this item was to investigate how semen donors deal with their condition in their social relationships: whether the subject is discussed or, on the contrary, whether it is kept secret.

Francisco, Luiz Cláudio and Ivan have never disclosed their status as semen donors. Francisco perceives his wife and her family as prejudiced people who, for this reason, would not accept his attitude. Therefore, maintaining absolute anonymity keeps him away from possible conflicts.

Luiz Cláudio told his close friends and family (parents and sisters) about his choice and experience with semen donation. However, he explained the subject using the figure of a colleague, who had been placed as the protagonist of the story, just to find out the opinions of the group. Since the opinions were unfavourable, the interviewee chose to hide his experience.

Ivan keeps his sperm donation hidden from his circle of friends and relatives, solely and exclusively because he received this advice from the semen bank, and he intends to keep his word. However, he would like to tell his loved ones, especially his son, whom he has as a partner, and who, in his opinion, would not only approve of his behaviour, but would probably become a donor too.

Milton, Tomaz and Edu shared the subject with those close to them: relatives and friends. The subjects reported that the majority of people do not approve of the attitude they have taken, but there are favourable opinions, generally from those who are not prejudiced, who are "open-minded". The reality observed by the three interviewees was similar to that seen by Luiz Cláudio in his social environment.

Edu reveals that one of his girlfriends was attracted to his *status* as a semen donor, associating the position with virility.

5.4.1.7 Semen users: heterosexuals, homosexuals, single people and older people

The majority of semen donors (Tomaz, Francisco, Ivan and Luiz Cláudio) are in favour of their gametes being used by all individuals who so wish: heterosexual and homosexual individuals and couples, as well as single people and the elderly of both sexes.

Milton and Edu are opposed to homosexuals as users of the semen they donate, because they are both against same-sex relationships. After delving deeper into the subject, Milton is in doubt as to whether he would exclude this class of men and women, saying that his refusal is restricted to "affected gays", who behave in a scandalous way, who cause scandals and shout in public, behaviour that he sees as reprehensible, which is not restricted to homosexuals, but extends to all people. In conclusion, according to the interviewee, individuals with these characteristics would certainly be excluded as recipients.

Edu thinks in terms of "biological truth", from what he says: "[...] man was made for woman and woman was made for man", which puts homosexuals in the position of deviants. When he thinks about "his child" being brought up by two mums or dads, he worries about the child's "head", which would probably be shaken by the social stigma surrounding homosexuals. The quote below illustrates this:

> But it's more of a social stigma, isn't it? Because society, most..., people have a father and a mother, and then the little child having two fathers or two mothers would be a bit strange at school, comparing people, everything, but it's more social. I think that, in terms of family, if you're brought up well, there isn't this... this part of the confusion, right? It's more in... what happens externally, right?

It's interesting to note that the kind of concern expressed by Edu is emphasised when the subject is the possibility of the life of a child who is biologically his, as can be seen here: "I don't think it's right. It's... and I also think it's complicated for a child to understand this, but... even more so my child. But if she has food on her plate to eat and if she has a good head on her shoulders in the future, I think she'll understand [...]".

Although he doesn't agree with homosexuality as a way of living a loving relationship, when he ponders the countless situations publicised daily by the media, involving aberrations, tragedies and evil, which affect all sorts of people, including children, Edu rethinks his initial position, opening up to the idea of homosexuals as possibly loving, caring and balanced fathers and mothers, which would give them the competence to bring up children. According to the interviewee:

> "[...] And so many people live with bigger problems than that. I don't think that's a problem. There are so many people who see their fathers murdered, their mothers raped, a lot of things that happen in life... I don't think having homosexual parents, and those things you mentioned (referring to the other users: heterosexuals, the elderly, and single people), is a problem."

Instead of taking a stance against homosexuals, Edu starts prioritising good parents as the ideal users of the gametes he donates, which is in line with Luiz Cláudio's opinion on the subject.

5.4.1.8 Child representation

The aim of this topic was to investigate how semen donors represent the figure of the child in their lives, what kind of space is offered to the offspring, what expectations are created, how they idealise fatherhood and so on.

The entire group of semen donors surveyed had representations of their child as a continuation of themselves, as a self-eternisation and also as a part of themselves. Some of the subjects (Tomaz and Luiz Cláudio) used the metaphor of the seed in an attempt to define the person who will descend from the donated sperm, as evidenced by Tomaz's statement when referring to the care that the recipient will be able to give to the child resulting from his donation: "The person has the conditions, went there, paid, did it, and is there looking after a little seed of mine".

Therefore, the father/donor will give part of himself for the constitution of the child, and the child will do the work of carrying on the physical and subjective characteristics (character, personality, humour, etc.) of his ancestor through his descendants who will come into existence, and so on and so forth.

One of the interviewees also raised another representation related to children, which refers to the pleasure of having the ability to give birth to a human being.

All the interviewees said they had a desire to experience fatherhood. However, the intensity of this desire varied among the group. Milton, Edu, Ivan and Francisco place the child at the highest level of their lives in terms of importance. According to the first subject, "the baby that will be born will be his fulfilment and that of his wife , because he is half of each of them". The transmission of self is so important to this subject that he is convinced that he will love the child that will be born more than his own wife, precisely because the child will carry within him half of the father (of the interviewee).

For Francisco, his son and his work are the most important things in his life, and his offspring is the most important thing, because he prioritises the professional area of his life, due to the fact that through his profession he will achieve financial stability which, in turn, will have to exist for the sake of the child, so that he can provide for all his needs.

Tomaz likes children. However, he doesn't intend to have a child, attributing his decision to the chaos that, in his view, is currently taking place in the world we live in. Although he wants his "little seed", produced by himself, to germinate and develop properly, he doesn't want to be its carer, nor would he want to know "its fruit", as this would change his status as an "independent person". On the contrary, he wants to transfer responsibility for his offspring to the recipient who chooses to fulfil this role.

As for Edu, he reveals that he likes children. He goes to children's parties, plays with them and they usually adore him. In addition, for the interviewee, producing children is the main mission of any human being's life. Everything else that is done, invented, built and lived represents the "extra hour" of a person's function in the world. This ideology of life has been equated since his childhood, when he began to experience intense conflicts and instabilities related to his own existence, in terms of the life/death cycle. Thus, for Edu, the descendants would play well-defined roles: they would promote the continuity of the ascendants, through the transmission of their genetic load and the life experiences of the genitor, while at the same time, the children would be ways of "circumventing" the inevitable and harsh reality of death.

Ivan is the only semen donor who has already experienced fatherhood. Now the father of a boy, a girl and a baby girl, he defines the experience of having children in much the same way as the other aspiring fathers. For the interviewee, having children had a very positive meaning and it was precisely the experience of this event that moved him to donate his gametes in order to help those individuals who lacked the ability to reproduce naturally. The quote illustrates the above:

> "[...] I would like someone to have the same feeling I had when I saw my son in the maternity ward. The paediatrician opened the little window and showed me: my son. [...] Man, I felt like I'd given birth to a child, that it's my sequence, that there's something inside it that's me, I don't know, it's going to stay in the world, a bit of me, you know? I will certainly go before him, and he will

> continue me, through things that are mine, but that are already part of him. That's how things are.

The interviewees were also asked how they understood the transmission of physical and subjective characteristics from ancestor to descendant. The vast majority attributed the transmission of all types of characteristics to genetic factors, as well as to the phenomenon of the social construction of the subject. Edu shares this idea, but he gives greater weight to learning in the environment, to the detriment of genetics. According to him, "the child is born zero in the head".

5.4.1.9 Destination of donated semen: collection, bank, recipient, IASD, pregnancy, birth, biological baby/child

Of all the interviewees, most (Milton, Tomaz, Francisco and Ivan) don't think about the fate of the material donated to the semen bank after donation. Milton understands the act objectively, and can be compared to the process of cryopreserving animal semen. Tomaz and Ivan prioritise the noble cause alone. Francisco doesn't attach any importance to the subject.

Edu likes to think of the circulation of his reproductive cells through the services provided by the semen bank. According to him, "the more, the better". On the other hand, the interviewee fears that his gametes will be used in illegal research that he believes exists. Such studies would be aimed at cloning human beings, hybridising humans and animals, creating specific organs or body parts for transplants, and so on.

Luiz Cláudio is happy for the guy who managed to realise his dream of patemidade/matemidade. For his part, he is happy to have been able to help his fellow man. He also reveals a personal satisfaction linked to the way he represents the CRT user in his imagination. For him, the people responsible for his biological child, due to his submission to assisted reproduction, are from higher social strata. As such, the child will probably have a wealthy, comfortable life, without deprivation, as well as receiving the best in terms of school education, being provided with what he himself could not offer.

5.4.1.10 Donor and the child generated by the donation

This topic was drawn up with the aim of finding out how the men interviewed deal with the child possibly generated through their sperm donated to the semen bank, who can be called their biological child.

Three interviewees (Milton, Edu and Luiz Cláudio) feel that they are the "fathers" of the children that came from their genetic material, even though these men are being kept away from any news about the fate of their donation. Of all of them, only Milton raised any questions about the matter with the semen bank. The others remained neutral.

The same individuals reported that they would like to meet the child and that they were curious about its physical characteristics. In addition, a certain degree of concern was identified on the part of the donors, which was associated with the well-being of the supposed "child", as well as the type of treatment it would be receiving.

Although he doesn't remain fixated on the subject of the results of his donations, Ivan also expresses a desire to get to know his descendants, and even to have some kind of closeness between them, which could extend to the important people in his life, such as his children and his mother.

Milton and Edu share Ivan's idea. Both subjects expressed their intention to take part in the child's life, helping in any way they could, giving guidance in times of doubt, accompanying them on outings and even providing financial support. However, Edu can't commit to this because he is going through a phase in which he is still establishing himself professionally and financially. The quotes below illustrate these statements:

> Honestly, if my children could know that I'm their father, I think it would be better. I'd like them to come to me at some point in their lives [...]. (Edu José)

> If [...] you gave me a list of the people who are with my children, I'd contact them one by one, and... I'd make a point of hanging out with the kids and everything. I'd even like to take part... the whole problem is that I'm still settling in, right? I'm not in a position to raise a child, or make a child for myself. So I think it would be a bit complicated for me to help raise the child, right? Even because the person wanted secrecy, it's... having the child was her decision and she didn't consult me, but I'd go there without a problem e.... (Edu José)

> As for meeting the child and it wanting to meet me, if it knew it was born from my semen, I wouldn't have anything against it, it's... on the contrary, I wouldn't have anything against it, and on the contrary, it would be a pleasure for me. I don't know, if something like that suddenly comes up, no, I'm not even worried about wanting to know that now, you know? But I have nothing against it. If she didn't have anything against it and her parents didn't have anything against it, I wouldn't have anything against it. I'd become friends, I'd introduce them to my children, they'd become friends. If, all of a sudden, I don't know, I'm no longer here on this earth and they're still friends, I have nothing against that. I think human beings have to be like that. People, no matter what, if they're brothers, if they're cousins, if they're only semen brothers, or whatever, people have to get along with each other, you know? Regardless of anything. (Ivan

Pessoa)

> To give you an idea... I don't think we'll ever get to know the child, do we? Is there any way of knowing them? There's no way, is there? [...] Ah, if the child wanted to meet me, I'd be happy to accept, no problem at all. I myself would like to know what it's like, right? A little speck of yours that came out... I'd like to know if you're well, if you're unwell, what you look like, right? People are always curious, right? (Luiz Cláudio)

> The contact with the semen bank was smooth, I asked all the questions I wanted and they were answered [...]. One of the questions I asked? One of the questions, I remember... if I... if I would know who the children would be... whether I wanted to or not, it's in our essence to want to know, right? If... if they were born, if their parents agreed... [...]. I think I'd like to know... about children. I'd like to... it's... I think to see, to see if they're being well looked after... I think that's it... to see the physical aspect as well, to see if they're not being... being mistreated, right? I think that's it... if... if I could, if the parents agreed, if you could contribute in some way, not financially, but in some other way that you could help. [..]) What kind of contribution would I like to make? Advice, if necessary, if he had any questions to clarify, that's all. If they had any doubts... I guess... like a parent, right? If your child has a question you try to answer it, if they ask for advice you give it, that's it. Now, if I had contact with the child and saw that they needed financial help? If I had the means, I would help, (silence). As I am, I would probably help. (Milton Jardim)

Francisco and Tomaz relate differently to the figure of their offspring generated by gametes that were donated at a specialised clinic, compared to the other subjects. Francisco doesn't consider himself to be the father of the child resulting from his semen. For him, paternity is developed through living together, in the exchanges established within the family. According to his explanation:

> "I think that the... the father is the one who creates, which I don't think is because my semen is there, that the one who's creating isn't going to be the father. I think he's a normal father, I don't think there's any problem [...] For the biological father I can't give zero, because if there was no semen there would be no child, so I give the father who creates... I give ten, or I give nine, so I can add up to ten (Francisco Sá)."

As such, the interviewee has no interest in meeting his biological son, but would agree to go and meet him if the child wanted him to, and with the authorisation of those responsible for him. The following quote illustrates this:

> "It's fine (to meet the child). But I'd like to talk to the family that's raising the child first. Because if he says, 'Oh, you'd better refuse because I'm afraid my child will like you more than... I'm the one who raised him, I'd rather you didn't meet him', I'll respect the father who made that choice. Now, if he says: 'No, that's fine with me', I will, I will want to meet him. I won't want to adopt him as a son, as nothing. I'll say: 'Oh, you have the genetic material, but all your philosophy, everything, everything you have to follow is from your father who raised you, I'm not your father (Francisco Sá)."

Unlike Francisco, Tomaz feels that his offspring are part of him and a continuation of him. However, throughout the interview, he made it clear or implied that he didn't feel in a position to take on the care necessary for the healthy development of a child. Possibly it was this reality, among others, that mobilised him to donate semen, since the context guarantees his genetic continuity, while at the same time transferring all the responsibilities required for the experience of fatherhood to those who choose to undergo ART. The issue is made clear when Tomaz discusses his relationship with money, as quoted below:

> [...] Because I personally can't afford to have a child. I have a good income, but I spend a lot... and... I have "n" financial problems. If a woman suddenly came knocking on my door, saying: 'Here, it's your child', then I don't know what I'd do, because I can't afford it... So I chose to donate, because someone will need it [...]. (Tomaz Lins)

One of the pieces of evidence that the figure of the child is important to Tomaz can be seen at a moment in the interview when he reveals that he would rather not meet the child that will be born from his semen, as this encounter would have an effect that would transform his current lifestyle. When asked about his desire to meet his anonymous offspring, the interviewee reveals the following: "I wouldn't like to, because if I meet the boy or girl, who I know is my child, then no... I'm not going to live like I do today. Knowing you have one is one thing; knowing who it is is something else (Tomaz)".

5.4.1.11 Donor as recipient

This topic aimed to find out how semen donors position themselves in relation to heterologous assisted reproduction, when put in the place of recipients.

The data collected points to the following results: half of the group (Tomaz, Francisco and Ivan) interviewed were in favour of the personal use of gametes cryopreserved in specialised clinics from an anonymous donor.

Tomaz Lins explains that not only would he agree to procreate using another man's sperm, but he would have that child as his own. He considers himself to be more "open" than most people are used to, and justifies the phenomenon on the basis of his sexual choice. Tomaz is bisexual.

Milton and Edu were initially resistant to the idea. Preliminarily, the former would prefer to resort to all possible infertility treatment resources. In the event of failure,

Milton's second option would be to adopt a child. The possibility of adoption was also mentioned by Edu and Luiz Cláudio. However, Luiz says that the final choice of which resource would make him a father would depend on the occasion and what he was going through.

For Edu, the use of the couple's own gametes is better for the dyad, as well as for the child itself. However, if the infertility issue wasn't resolved, since the child wouldn't be his biologically, he would prefer adoption, because the child to be adopted is waiting for his parents and needs a family to look after him, which would be more humane. According to the quotes:

Furthermore, the testimonies of the three agents: Milton, Edu and Luiz Cláudio pointed to the fact that, even if they were not in favour of the IASD, they would agree to procreate in this way in order to share their wives' wishes. If the woman wanted to experience pregnancy and/or if it was important for her to pass on her genes, as it is for Edu, their husbands would do everything possible to fulfil their wives' wishes. For, as Luiz Claudio explains: "You get married not to make yourself happy. You get married to make your wife happy".

In the case of reproduction using the technique of heterologous artificial insemination, Milton and Francisco would make a point of choosing the material based on the phenotypical similarity between the social father and the semen donor.

5.4.1.12 Religiosity

The aim of this item was to find out about the agents' training and current religious experience, in order to identify possible links between the theme and the question that serves as the basis for this work.

All six subjects had some kind of religious background during their childhood. Nowadays, the type of relationship maintained with transcendence varies between the agents.

Tomaz is an evangelical, but not a regular or fervent practitioner. He occasionally attends church and, at the time of the interview, he hadn't been to services for a long time.

For a long time, Milton dedicated himself to reading about Allan Kardec's spiritism, and until then he claimed to be an adherent of that branch of religion. However, when he "immersed" himself in the subject, he found insurmountable inconsistencies that led him to distance himself from "Kardecism". Nowadays, Milton calls himself a Catholic and attends church occasionally, where he feels in tune, both in theory and in practice.

Luiz Cláudio calls himself "a Catholic who is a bit distorted by life", which he defines as different from "the one who is really Catholic, who follows the rules and goes to church every week". He considers himself a non-practising Catholic, who accepts getting to know other religious modalities.

Milton, Tomaz and Luiz Cláudio say that they have a religious conviction. However, they are the owners of their own thoughts, which at times may diverge from the precepts of their respective religions.

Edu and Francisco introduced themselves as atheists. However, the individuals experience atheism in different ways. Both subjects had attended various religions and spiritualist philosophies, which were insufficient to satisfy and convince them.

During the meeting we had, Francisco showed himself, from start to finish, as someone who understands life as something limited to matter, the concrete, the tangible. At no point did he express feeling the need for a religious life, nor did he give any information suggesting a relationship with some kind of divinity, or even the possibility of the existence or continuity of the spirit when the body doesn't exist, or even the desire to reflect on the subject, even though he was brought up in a devoutly Catholic family. The quote illustrates the point:

> My mum always said: 'You've got to find a religion! Go to church with me. Go to mass one Sunday! I'd say: 'No, I don't really believe... in... in that! I went for a short time, two, three months. I saw that it didn't add anything to my life and.... I didn't go along with it. I said: 'No. There's no point! [...] I think I'm more of an atheist. I think atheist is a very strong word. But I think I'm more of an atheist than anything else. Like not believing in anything at all. What I haven't seen, I don't believe in." (Francisco)

When asked how he interprets life and death, Francisco says: "It's dead, it's over and I've never stopped to try to go deeper. According to him, "there's no continuity, no aspect of the soul, nothing. No, it's over, the next one comes".

Edu has a different religious background compared to Francisco. Based on our "encounter", as described in the material in sub-section 5.3.2, I think that Edu has not yet defined himself in religious or spiritual terms, and I would venture to say that the issue in question seems to act as the axis of his existence, mobilising his emotions and thoughts, defining him in personal and professional terms, and his entire life trajectory. His disquiet about the subject, which began in his early years, still seems to be latent.

It's worth pointing out that, during the three hours we spent together: walking down the street, inside my car and at my home, the only time the interviewee tried to get into my personal life was when we discussed the subject of this topic, when he asked about a sticker from a Zen Buddhist spiritualist brotherhood that was fixed to the top of the rear window of my car. The way Edu questioned me was curious: abrupt, emphatic, inquisitive. There was such force and speed in his subsequent questions that they left me no room to answer or think. It was as if they had been held back for a long time. It was as if he was looking for the answers to his own questions in my answers. The ones with which Edu wants to silence the fear of death that has mobilised him for so long.

Although he calls himself an atheist, Edu says he is "open to various religious beliefs and practices". He usually goes to the Catholic church with his grandmother; he attends the "Gospel at Home" spiritual service held weekly by his mother at her home; and he has become interested in the philosophy of the Mormons, which he translates as corporatist.

The donors are also eclectic in religious terms: Ivan and Luiz
Claudio.

Tomaz, Milton, Ivan and Luiz Cláudio believe in a God and this entity is understood by them as the creator of the universe and everything that belongs to it, including human beings, to whom they owe respect and devotion.

With regard to semen donation, Milton, Tomaz and Luiz Cláudio say that they imagine their religions are against the practice.

The agents who showed that they were motivated to donate semen by religious aspects were Milton, Ivan and Edu.

5.4.1.13 Donor and some questions about "race"

Information on "race" was collected in the first part of the script: personal data. However, the data collected was limited to the subjects' racial self-classification, since the subject of "race" is not part of the objectives of this study.

According to the results, four respondents classified themselves as "white". The non-white individuals found it more difficult to define themselves in terms of "race". One of them (Francisco) called himself "brown", or "light brown". The last (Luiz Cláudio) answered as follows: "I don't know what to tell you about that question, because there are blondes and brunettes in my family and I have a bit of European blood, because there is a bit of Portuguese and French in my family, from my grandparents".

As the subject seemed to generate a certain amount of discomfort in the interviewee, I opted for generalisation. I then went on to talk about Brazil's racial characteristics of miscegenation, which reproduce his own reality. Based on this, I asked the interviewee to categorise himself in terms of "race", using a single word, to which Luiz Cláudio replied as follows: "I believe that I'm not a legitimate black person, because my family has all kinds of ethnicities and my parents are light skinned. So I class myself as brown.

The two mestizo agents in the group studied, in my opinion, who were close to the dark side, were precisely those who showed a certain instability in their racial self-classification. Luiz Cláudio emphasised the existence of a conflict regarding his racial characteristics

black, which seems to differ from her "light" parents and her European ancestry, as mentioned above. In this respect, it was interesting to note that his visible African ancestry was not even mentioned. As for Francisco, the interviewee would have tended towards whitening by calling himself "light brown". This phenomenon seems to reflect Brazil's racial characteristics, based on the false idea of racial democracy and the ideology of whitening.

Studies on the subject of "race" point to the issue of the false notion of racial democracy that exists in Latin American countries, especially in Brazil, where miscegenation on a biological level and miscegenation on a sociological level have been confused. These notions about racial democracy were formulated by intellectuals based on pre-existing ideas proclaiming the superior benevolence of the slave system in their respective societies. In addition, this racial myth emphasised miscegenation as an indicator of racial tolerance and apologia da mestiçagem. In the Brazilian case in particular, these notions have been embraced by the state, making the situation official, which has been incorporated into common sense, resulting in the conception of race relations as equal and non-conflicting, which in fact cover up the reality of racism and social inequalities based on "race", in which white subjects are superimposed on non-white subjects (mestizos and blacks).

As a result of racism and interracial social inequalities, the Brazilian reality has produced an ideology of whitening, which has been incorporated by non-white individuals and, on the other hand, the latter have a low self-esteem linked to their Afro-descent. According to Carlos Hasenbalg, a scholar on the subject,

> [...] one can point to an experience reported by several researchers about their fieldwork. This is the situation of initial embarrassment and awkwardness created when the researcher asks their interviewees or informants about their colour and the situations of racial discrimination they have experienced. The

> embarrassment, felt particularly by poorly educated interviewees, is already an indication that people are not used to speaking naturally about issues relating to race relations (HASENBALG, 1996, p. 243).

As for the ideology of whitening, its assimilation by non-white people has become a mechanism for the psychosocial insertion of black people into a world dominated by whites. The notion of whitening is sometimes seen as the internalisation of white cultural models by the black segment, implying the loss of its African *ethos*, and sometimes it is defined by authors as the process of "whitening" of the Brazilian population, recorded by official censuses and statistical forecasts from the late 19th and early 20th centuries, being one of the modalities of Brazilian racism (DOMINGUES, 2002).

5.4.1.14 Donor profile

All those interviewed have the profile of a donor of human material, and/or function in life in a generous and altruistic way.

Milton, Tomaz, Edu, Ivan and Luiz Cláudio are regular blood donors. Francisco doesn't donate because he doesn't have the time, but he would endeavour to do so if it were necessary for someone else. He points out that he prioritises helping others, but does so if he doesn't want to harm himself.

As well as being a blood and organ donor, Milton often distributes his belongings (clothes, shoes, etc.) to the needy.

Edu didn't declare himself an "organ donor" on his identification documents (ID and driving licence) because he didn't trust unknown people very much. Otherwise, in the event of a fatality, his death could be hastened by the medical field, due to other interests. Based on the above, the individual says that he thinks first of himself and then of others, which seems to be a difficulty in accepting himself as belonging to the sphere of altruism. It's interesting to note that, even though Edu thinks of himself as self-interested, he reveals that he left a signed letter in his own handwriting authorising his relatives to donate his organs, in the event that he becomes brain-dead, so that other people can benefit from them in transplants.

5.4.1.15 Motivation for participating in the research

Edu was motivated to take part in this research in order to "publicise what he thinks and wants", to expose himself, as this could help him to be found in the future by his children born from donated gametes.

The other five interviewees took part in this study to collaborate for altruistic purposes.

5.4.1.16 Experience with sperm donation at a semen bank

Based on the association between the material collected during a visit to the semen bank in 2008 and the data collected in the field study, sperm donation takes place in the following way: initially, the prospective donor contacts the bank to obtain information on the subject, which usually happens by *email* and/or telephone. The clinic usually responds quickly, providing instructions related to screening, which is the phase in which the man undergoes a medical consultation, serological and chromosomal tests, and sperm collection, for which the individual must have completed a four-day period of sexual abstinence. These screening stages don't necessarily take place in the same order or on the same day. Once the *quarantine* period has passed, the candidate returns to the bank to repeat the sperm collection and tests, becoming a de facto donor if the results are satisfactory[30] .

The aim of this topic was to find out how the group that donates sperm to a specialised bank dealt with the experience of semen donation, as well as other aspects related to the practice.

The results obtained from the data collected revealed a division of opinions regarding the group's perception of the sperm donation experience, as well as the existence of a certain ambiguity in Ivan Pessoa's testimony.

For three subjects (Milton, Francisco and Ivan), everything they had to experience to become registered donors at the semen bank was quite natural. The journey to the clinic, arriving there, contact with the reception, the bank's premises, completing the screening stages, collecting the gametes, delivering the material, leaving the establishment, returning, in short, all the procedures required to donate semen were always experienced spontaneously by the interviewees. When they came into contact with the clinic, Francisco and Milton explained that they felt welcomed by the professionals, with whom they had room to ask questions, give answers and make decisions about whether or not to donate. According to Francisco: "I had no problems. Everyone was very professional and kind. I saw everything very naturally.

[30] The process is discussed in more detail in the first chapter of this thesis.

The other subjects experienced the process of donating sperm as very difficult, especially during their first contact with the bank, as Tomaz revealed: "I had to break down a barrier!".

One caveat. On the dates of the interviews with these individuals, Luiz Cláudio had only visited the clinic once, Tomaz had made two donations, and Edu has been donating semen for seven years. As such, the difficulties experienced by the last interviewee have changed over time. However, he still reported conflict-producing situations.

Due to his busy working day, Luiz Cláudio had to schedule a Saturday morning to complete the screening of donation candidates. He reported being overwhelmed by intense doubts as the scheduled date approached. On the day, on the way to the semen bank, the agent was crossed by feelings of inconstancy and fear, as can be seen in his statement: "So then I went. I got in the way, I was like, I'm going, I'm not I'm going, I'm going, I'm not going...".

The feelings of fear and insecurity mentioned are associated with various factors. Firstly, the visit to the clinic specialising in the storage of male reproductive cells promotes "real" contact with a universe that, until then, had only been known virtually, via the Internet, in other words, it represents the "materialisation" of an act that had only been experienced at the level of fantasy. As well as migrating from the virtual to the face-to-face, completing the screening stage introduces the subject to a new reality, which can generate feelings of insecurity and fear. According to Luiz Cláudio's account of his first trip to the semen bank: "[...] it was a unique experience. It was something new, because I'd never really done anything like this before. I went from theory to practice.

Secondly, in general, someone's stay in a certain place always implies the possibility of casual encounters with people they know, and this can also happen in the immediate vicinity of the place. In this sense, for a donor who wants to remain anonymous, going to a semen bank represents an imminent danger, since being in a company that offers sperm storage and supply services for assisted reproduction "speaks for itself" about a fact that should be kept secret. In the case of the bank where the interviewees are registered, the issue requires greater care. Despite having a discreet façade, the clinic is located at the back of the ground floor of a commercial building with a lot of passers-by. Luiz Cláudio's statement illustrates this: "[...] At first I was a bit embarrassed because I didn't know who I was going to see there, something new, everyone knows why you're there".

Thirdly, the supply of one's own gametes to a semen bank has significant consequences, which can weigh heavily on the donor when the act is carried out. Luiz Cláudio reports that he felt overwhelmed by a state of insecurity during the journey from his home to the clinic, when he reflected on the results that could come from donating his semen and the changes that these could cause in his life. According to the subject: "Semen donation has results, which is a child of your own, a child who, I don't know what it's going to be like? Then, on the way, I thought, well, I'm so happy with my life...".

Tomaz recounts another event resulting from his fear of the consequences of donating semen. According to Tomaz, after bottling the collected sperm and delivering the container to the right place, an intense feeling of remorse came over him, resulting in him wanting to give up his initial intention, which was eased by thinking about the altruism involved in the situation . The quote below illustrates this:

> So, after the act was done, after closing that little door and leaving the consulting room, I felt a pang of remorse, a weight [...]. It was like that at the time, it gave me a... it made me want to go back and say 'Give it to me! But no, it was something like that, a snap in a minute, even less, it was a, a very quick thing, but right afterwards it was a relief, something like... I did a good thing. I did a good thing." (Tomaz)

At another point in the interview, Tomaz revealed that he was very worried about another possible consequence of donating semen: his responsibility for the child generated using his sperm. According to his account: "I was really worried, because I said... can you imagine, then someone comes along and... I don't know, takes my details, turns up at the house saying: 'Oh, it's your child!' 'No, I never did anything to you!' 'No, but it's yours and I want alimony!' (laughs)".

According to Tomaz's testimony, contact with the semen bank and the experience of the sperm donation process were very difficult, and another aspect was related: the perception of the practice as something "technical and cold", which would have caused him both embarrassment and fear. The emotions were such that they affected the collection of the material and, consequently, the results of the spermogram carried out by Tomaz. For this reason, the interviewee was asked by the bank to repeat the semen collection, due to the low concentration of sperm in his diagnostic test. The following quote illustrates this:

> [The semen donation process] was a bit embarrassing, because I'd never done it before, you know? When you arrive, you're in a spare room, you don't see anyone's face, just... the... a... nurse, I don't know if it's the nurse. She arrives, then guides you into that little room, there are all the instructions inside the little room, there's a video, there's a DVD, to help you, if you need it, there's a magazine. It was difficult. I went twice. The first time, she sent me the count, but it wasn't enough, because I was... I was embarrassed. I wanted to do it, but

> I was embarrassed at the time. Let's say I'd had *a blowjob*, you know? (...) So much so that ....I believe
> I couldn't make the donation on the first day because I was a bit embarrassed, scared. It was a lot of fear.

Edu José, a semen donor for seven years, now feels adapted to the routine intrinsic to this type of voluntary practice. However, his first experiences with the specialised bank involved difficulties and embarrassment, just like those mentioned by the other agents. During the time he has been donating semen, he has had to repeat all the tests required of a prospective donor, every year. Every month, Edu has been asked by the bank to provide a new sample of the material (semen), which only happens every two months, due to his professional commitments.

The investigated agent expressed a high degree of concern about the image of the individual who donates sperm, constantly focussing on his own status as a donor. He says he perceives an "atmosphere" both inside the clinic and in the *hallway* of the building, where there is a guardhouse, building staff and people circulating or waiting on benches. For Edu, the "atmosphere" present in those environments seems to reveal the existence of a stigma attached to the figure of the semen donor, which would be confirmed by the behaviour of others.

As the semen bank is located at the back of the building's *hallway*, to get to the entrance of the clinic, the individual has to walk a few metres and must pass through the guardhouse, even though there is no need to register to visit the bank. As he walks along this route, Edu often notices stares that accompany him all the time, something that has been repeated since the time when the semen bank belonged *to the Albert Einstein Hospital.* According to his account: "[...] When you go in, people stare at you. There was also a centre at *Einstein*, and when you went into the room, everyone would be there, and here in the building too, people would be looking at you [...]".

As for the stigma associated with the donor within the semen bank itself, Edu points to facts related to the treatment of the group. On arrival, the sperm collector is usually welcomed by a member of staff. At the end of the process, the donor always leaves alone. The following quote makes the point:

> É... The staff, when you arrive, they welcome you, don't they? They arrive and say: 'Hi, I don't know what'! Then when you leave, nobody looks at you, right? You leave straight away, there's no-one there. So it's kind of a thing, isn't it? When you leave, nobody wants to greet you, take your hand, say 'bye'. There's no kissing or anything (Edu).

As well as Edu, Ivan Pessoa had also felt discomfort associated with going out alone after the donation, as well as realising the existence of the aforementioned "climate" permeating the relationships maintained with the semen bank. However, Ivan names the "climate" using other expressions: mist and *fog*. Unlike Edu, he doesn't consider outside gazes to be relevant, thus confining the fog to the clinic where his gametes are supplied. In line with the above, Ivan expresses the following: "I don't give a damn what anyone thinks or says about me".

Ivan Pessoa identifies aspects of the fog in the way the semen bank is run, in general, which he interprets as a "[...] limitation on the part of the staff who work there, the owner of the clinic, the management itself. They create a fog, a haze that doesn't need to be there". The interviewee criticises certain attitudes at the bank: the excessive reserve in dealing with the subject of semen donation; the lack of naturalness in dealing with the subject; the reinforcement of the invisibility of the practice and the practitioner; the lack of campaigns aimed at gamete donation, including and especially within the bank itself; the pedantry resulting from a self-perception of superiority, due to the fact that they work in favour of conception; the neglect of the donor who, in his view, performs the noblest act. The quote below complements the above:

> What's this mist for? Nothing, nothing. I think it should be *lighter*. That's no sin! There should be more... there should be a lot of campaigning on the walls asking for help, showing that this is the place. I think the campaign should start there on the walls, or on leaflets, in vows, with the words: 'Become a volunteer, I don't know what! I'd be the first to take the material and leave it at the club, I'd distribute it in the streets, something like that. People seem to be a bit limited, I don't know. They should get rid of the taboo in their heads.

Ivan continued:

> What does the taboo have to do with anything? I don't know. I think they work with a human area that... I don't know. There's a little bit of feeling like a king, I think. Of saying: 'We bring human beings into the world! I think they're a bit pedantic. I've always had that idea. They have this feeling of being kind of divine... They're not doing us any favours! They're not doing you any favours! I think the noblest attitude is that of the giver, regardless of whether it's me, or whether they want confetti on me. I don't want anything, but people there only regulate, they're full of reservations.

The bank's behaviour of welcoming donors on arrival and only escorting them as far as the entrance to the sperm collection room may be indicating care rather than the opposite. If we think that the extraction of semen involves masturbation/orgasm/ejaculation, with which various symbolisms are associated, the presence of someone at the time of departure may embarrass some individuals, as was seen in the testimony of Tomaz, who felt that contact with the bank at all stages of donation was very difficult. According to the interviewee: "The whole thing was very difficult for me, I felt very scared. After I left the room I didn't see anyone else and it was good, I felt better. It would have been terrible if one of those nurses had turned up to say goodbye to me". On the other hand, on the day I visited the clinic, I felt very welcomed by everyone and, as soon as the interview was finalised, the director of the semen bank kindly led me to the door, where we said a fond farewell.

In order to remove the "ghosts" of stigma from the contact between the donor and the semen bank, some devices could be used. For example, a resource that might satisfy all the subjects could be the adoption of a live voice system that broadcasts a thank you and farewell message on behalf of the semen bank as the donor leaves the collection room and heads for the clinic exit. In addition, there could be a face-to-face farewell, if the donor prefers.

According to half of the interviewees, another aspect that they considered important in the practice of sperm donation, and which is closely linked to the themes presented here, refers to the environment in which the material is collected. This is an area made up of an anteroom, a living room and a bathroom. In this last room there are all the instructions for the collection, in printed form: initial and final asepsis, collection, storage of the material, delivery, etc. In the main room there is: a sofa, a television with cable channels, a VCR, a DVD *player* and various pornographic films and magazines. In front of the television there is a "little door" that must be opened when the vial for storing the semen is handed over and, from then on, the individual is free to leave the clinic. The comments made by the donors were based on the following elements: pornography, ejaculation, pleasure, semen donation, stigma, science, the laboratory, technology, commerce, the donor's social stratification, and others.

With regard to the collection environment, one of the interviewees (Edu) mentioned experiencing a type of antagonism related to pornographic resources, aimed at stimulating men; the objective with sperm donation, which is to help resolve certain cases of infertility; and the intermediation of the semen bank, which is based on medical and technological areas.

According to Edu: "It's strange. You're watching the 'big porn' there, then suddenly you finish, close the jar and give it to the headmistress and they're all there, all the equipment. Then you close that little window. It's really strange, but I'm used to it. I've been doing it for a long time.

For him, it wouldn't be necessary to have all those pornographic resources in the sperm collection environment, "for the sake of the person's education". In his opinion, "looking at the ethical side of the business, it would be better if there wasn't" (the amount of pornography on site), because the reality in question would create a distortion in relation to the function of semen donation and the donor's own intention, generating stigma, already mentioned.

Returning to the question of sperm donor stigma, Edu explains that the prejudice in which the agent and the practice would be inserted refers mainly to the way in which the material supplied is extracted: through masturbation, a reality that seems to place this type of donation in a place of tare equivalence, and the donor in the position of a sexual deviant.

During our meeting, Edu emphasised that several people with whom he has close relationships (relatives and friends) and who were involved in his life choice, often "make fun" of his status as a semen donor. During socialising or festivities, the interviewee is often called a "wanker" by his loved ones. Therefore, according to his personal analysis, the looks that accompany him to the clinic and the treatment he receives at the semen bank are intrinsically linked to the "masturbator" image associated with the sperm donor. As a way of elucidating this reflection, an extract from the interview with Edu is reproduced below:

> Ana Paula: [...] It's interesting because with you this question is becoming very strong, that there's something marginal about giving. I don't know if I can use that word.
>
> Edu José: Yes, you can!
>
> Ana Paula: When you enter the building and everyone's looking, what do they think?
>
> Edu José: Well, you're going to have a wank, aren't you?
>
> Ana Paula: The problem is the "wank".
>
> Edu José: It's the "wank". You go and have a wank and everyone's like: "Oh, the guy's a wanker, I don't know what...". Just like my friends also make fun of him, right? But that's not it, you know? It's the way you get it out, you know? So, if I need to do what I need to do, I'll do it. It's not like I go there and stay there because there's a new video, because there's a new magazine, because the place is cool. I do whatever I want at home, right? But it's... people think, you know? That's what stays in my head.

In the not many national socio-anthropological studies that mention masturbation, the practice is circumscribed to transgression, as a reflection of the social constructions relating to sexuality in so-called Western societies, which seems to justify the notion of semen donor as synonymous with "wanker", as seen in Edu's statement.

For anthropologist Richard Parker, it is the erotic dimension of sexuality that particularises sexual culture in Brazil, thought of as a whole or as a relatively homogenous whole. Within the erotic frame of reference, according to Parker, the body and genitals, in particular, are seen as instruments of pleasure, rather than markers of power, all depending on the context. More than anything, it is the notion of transgression that defines the culture of eroticism in our contemporary culture. As such, masturbation, anal intercourse and oral sex "precisely because of the numerous prohibitions that surround them, fit perfectly into the transgressive structure of eroticism - a world of 'dirty', horniness and pleasure". (PARKER, 1994, p. 12-13).

Luna (2007), when discussing sterility in the context of the technologies of procreation, cites anthropologist Françoise Héritier's (1984) analyses of the misconduct sanctioned by sterility, which are seen as acts of transgression that break the cosmic order and balance, and are related to the rules of kinship. Such acts of transgression imply three types of crossing: of generations, of blood and of genders. Self-sexuality or masturbation represents a type of gender crossing.

> [...] These are acts of transgression that disrupt the cosmic order and its equilibrium.
> [...] contamination between the male and female genders is avoided in the practices of homosexuality, self-sexuality (masturbation), and between other genders that must be kept separate [...] (LUNA, 2007, p. 181).

In Ivan Pessoa's case, other contrasting feelings emerged from his contact with the semen bank's premises, where there is a "little door" that divides two spaces: the collection room and the clinic's laboratory.

On his first visit to the semen bank, when he was taken to the specific collection room, Ivan was instructed as follows: after depositing the material in the appropriate vial, he was to hand it in at the "little door" mentioned above. Driven by curiosity, he opened the door, before the steps he still had to go through.

On the other side of the "little door" is the bank's laboratory, where treatments are carried out to analyse the concentration and motility of the spermatozoa and the subsequent process of freezing the material. To carry out the semen culture stages, specific state-of-the-art equipment is used, as well as a team of specialised technical professionals. This means that there are people on site, including women, handling test tubes, flasks, containers, diluents, solutions, pipettes, *beckers*, microscopes, cylinders, *freezers* and so on. This means that through the "little door" there is all the human technological apparatus that makes up the sperm analysis and cryopreservation laboratory in operation.

The scene outside the "little door" had an impact on Ivan, bringing up conflicts related to semen donation. Even so, he managed to finalise the sperm collection process and deliver the bottled material to the stipulated location, according to him, because he was "open-minded", something that probably wouldn't be possible for men with opposite characteristics. Let's look at the quote below:

> She gave me the bottle to collect it and said: 'Look, when you've finished collecting it, it's... there's something inside, you'll see it right in front of the television, you'll see a little door, so you can open that little door and hand it in'. I thought that 'you can hand it in' meant that it was left somewhere, something like that. I'm *not bothered* about that. In reality, I opened that little door, even before I made the collection, to see what it was there, right? And in reality, here's the thing... the laboratory is there. The girls are working there, test tubes, I don't know what, over there. So, in reality, when you do the collection, you know? And then, when the material is ready, you open that little door and hand it over to the girl. I think there are people who collect semen, I don't know what, and don't open that little door. If the guy opened it first, you know? Some people don't hand it over. Now, there are people who, I think, deep down, deep down, I think they should open it and close it, and leave it there and go away, and never come back. (Ivan)

The subject's testimony about his experience was truncated throughout. Even though we walked together towards a deeper understanding of the issue, his thoughts were "chopped up", but it was possible to extract some meanings from them.

Ivan had highlighted the existence of conflicts that seemed to be related to the same universe mentioned by Edu. It was the same world seen through a different prism.

Following the clues provided, for the agent, being a voluntary sperm donor and having contact with the technological area of the clinic produces: "impact", "stagnation", leaves the man feeling "bored", gives a sensation of "ice on the body", provokes "indignation", whose reactions are generated by factors that I will try to describe.

On his first contact with the post-door enclosure, before collecting the semen, Ivan saw a laboratory where female professionals were working. In the second contact with the same place, after collecting the sperm, the individual opened the "little door" and handed over the bottle. After saying thank you and goodbye, the donor closed the "little door", left the collection room, went downstairs, passed the reception desk and left the bank, without having seen anyone else. According to Ivan, being in the position of donor, the clinic acted carelessly towards the volunteer, because, in his opinion, the existence of the aforementioned "little door" and the possibility it creates: contact between donor and laboratory, "is improper and unnecessary, or even unfriendly".

During the interview, the subject made some revelations about the conflicts mentioned, which were linked to the taboo and symbolism of semen. Firstly, handing over the material collected in a specific bottle and bagged in a transparent wrapping makes the seminal fluid visible. The visibility of the material produces embarrassment because, in Western societies, semen is associated with sex, and sex is associated with taboo. On the other hand, the attitude of handing sperm over to a laboratory makes it similar to other substances of different importance, such as urine, which has a purifying action and is disposable, compared to semen, which carries the individual's genetic load and produces a new being. Thus, urine and semen carry asymmetrical symbolic charges (impurity vs. life), which are interpreted according to the wider social system, as discussed by Mary Douglas (1966) in her work Purity and *Danger*.

The two realities: the visibility of semen and the perception of similarity between sperm and other substances of lesser value would have been conflict-producing factors for Ivan Pessoa, as can be seen in the following quote:

> [...] it's just that in reality, when you hand it to the person, it's already in a hermetically sealed test tube, with a plastic lid and then you put it in a bag, zip it up and that's how you hand it over, you know? There's no coloured bag to cover anything, and you feel like you're handing over urine, right? And in reality it's semen, it's sperm. So there's milky semen, there's something that creates... it shouldn't be. I think this leads to someone not being a donor, you know?

I now propose that we go back a little. Between the two contacts through the "little door", Ivan proceeded to collect the sperm. To do this, the individual needs to reach a state of sexual arousal, which is stimulated by erotic magazines and films, in which images of nudity of the female body in erotic scenes are abundantly displayed, and it is from these that the man is able to extract the material, when he reaches the point of ejaculation. Immediately after this phase, the subject opens the little door, when he realises that there are other elements associated with the act: the laboratory and the young professionals who work there.

In recounting this experience, Ivan expresses deep indignation at the way the semen bank works, especially with regard to the criteria adopted for the stages following the collection of the material. This would turn the individual volunteer into a mere sperm supplier, and the reproductive cells into products to be industrialised and marketed. According to the aforementioned:

> Look, that's... you collect it and give it there, isn't it... isn't there an expression that says 'I'm what, a donor'?what, a sperm donor?donor? Understand? So, there are people who
> ends up saying: 'I came here thinking that a noble donation, but I'm just a sperm donor, that's all'. Got it?

A from theabove, Ivan formulates some hypotheses. Firstly, the indignationfelt was contained in him, and so it must bewith the other donors, because of the

their level of socialisation and their belonging to higher social strata, which would turn them into more restrained people. Whereas other men who are less educated, less enlightened, not as well-trained as he is, and who belong to lower social classes, would probably react to the situation in question in a more instinctive and aggressive way, above all due to the fact that they are part of a Latin culture where machismo reigns supreme, as well as the fact that donation also has connotations of sexuality. Let's look at the following quote:

> I didn't see it that way, but human beings, especially Latinos, are very macho. There are so many people on the street who make fun of girls, who say this, that, you have these things. After all, it's not blood you're donating, it's semen you're donating, which in reality is linked by a large section of the population, which is a sexist section, to... the sexual relationship you have with a woman. Then all of a sudden you see someone, any girl, grab the thing out of your hand, even deliberately, all of a sudden, the guy would bump into her hand, or all of a sudden the guy would tug on it... because there's a side to it, right? There's a sexual connotation, right? You know? I think. (Ivan)

Another supposition put forward by Ivan is the suspicion that the selection of semen donors is based on the social levels to which the men are linked. Furthermore, this same reason would justify the existence of so few individuals registered at the clinic. The following quote illustrates this:

> [...] Now, you see that they qualify the donors, right? In a way that would be a modest guy, a guy who had a bit more study, who wouldn't go, right? Because if they were all donors, any type of donor there was in the clinic, they wouldn't put it like that. Because they don't know what the person's reaction will be. They don't know if, all of a sudden, the guy is going to be there, turn on the television, all of a sudden know what's going on over there, because he's seen it before, 'Well, I can't do it. You can't come here, can you? I don't know. If they had donors from all sorts of walks of life, they wouldn't risk something like this, you know? That's why I don't think they have that many donors either.

The interviewee raises another issue. As soon as he feels he has been reduced to a mere "sperm donor", the semen he donates is no longer linked to the sphere of the gift, but to the sphere of the market, which is exposed by the luxury of the semen bank's facilities and decor. According to her statement:

> [...] But the thought you have afterwards is: 'Well, I'm a sperm donor, I'm here as a volunteer and they treat me like this? Man, they're making a fortune out of this! People think, don't they? I think it's natural for human beings. It's a sumptuous clinic, they must make a *lot* of money here, and they treat me like

that? I went there and well, you know? When I walked in... "sperm donor!" (Ivan)

From the data collected in the interviews with gamete donors, and presented here in this topic, some axes of analysis could be highlighted for discussion, such as the representations of semen in different types of society; the question of taboo in the practice in focus, or even the relationship between sex and gender identities in the donation process, for example. However, based on the object of study chosen for this research, I intend to prioritise an issue arising from the "complaints" of the men studied, which converge on a single point: the dehumanisation of the gift that exists in semen donation. Based on the above, the question arises: why does the gift that donors give to the semen bank have to be transformed into something of less value? Why does the gift have to be turned into a product? Why do the men who provide sperm to semen banks have to be subjected to so many constraints? Why isn't semen donation humanised?

Section 5.4.2, on analysing the category of this study, will discuss the issues in question.

5.4.1.17 Final thoughts from the agents

This topic was addressed at the end of each meeting and was intended to provide space for any comments that the agents felt were relevant to the topic under investigation and that might not have been included in the script used in the interviews, or even if they had been exposed but not sufficiently discussed by the interviewees. Only Edu José and Tomaz Lins presented final considerations .

Edu explained that, in fact, he has no difficulty whatsoever in disclosing his identity when donating semen. In other words, as a donor, he has chosen not to conceal the reality of his life's goal, which is to procreate, from his relationships. However, during his visits to the semen bank, he often feels that he is being watched, as was shown in the previous topic on the *agents' experience of donating reproductive cells.* In this sense, it was important for Edu to say that he would like the specialised clinic to offer more privacy to the men who come there to voluntarily collect the material, and Ivan Pessoa mentioned the same thing.

Furthermore, Edu points out that, as his life mission is based on procreation, it would be possible for him to have a sexual relationship with a woman who wanted to become pregnant, if she did not wish to undergo assisted reproduction treatments.

Tomaz ended his interview by explaining that the subject of gamete donation should be more widely publicised in the media, whose stories could prioritise the reality of the facts rather than sensationalism. In his opinion, soap operas tend to misrepresent the subject, causing concern for those who have lived through this type of experience, such as donors, recipients, the children they give birth to and all those involved in the situation in one way or another.

In addition, the interviewee says that the way in which these children were conceived should be known to him, as well as being exposed to family members and family friends. In his view, "the 'guy' who lives through the process of conception, birth and the child's development is the child's real father". According to Tomaz, "the truth always has to be told, so as not to cause conflicts in the future". However, if this is the donor's wish, the individual's identity should be kept anonymous.

Furthermore, according to Tomaz's testimony, all people who experience procreation with donated gametes should undergo a psychological or psychiatric assessment beforehand, as well as monitoring by the same specialists, in order to prevent conflicts, suffering and maladjustments that can arise when experiencing the situation, as the following quote shows:

> Anyone who has been involved in semen donation or egg donation, whether it's the donor, the mother, the father, the family members or the child, should see a psychologist or a psychiatrist to see if they're able to live with this kind of thing, if they're prepared for it. It was a mistake not to have seen a psychologist. I thought I would have." (Tomaz Lins)

Below are the tables listing the subjects and their respective personal details.

Personal details of the semen donors interviewed:

SUBJECT	AGE	AGE 1*. DONATION	TIME AS A DONOR	PROFESSION
MILTON JARDIM	28 YEARS	27 YEARS	1 YEAR	LAWYER
TOMÁZ LINS	31 YEARS	IDEM	6 MONTHS	STUDENT OF ACCOUNTING
EDÚJOSÉ	28 YEARS	21 YEARS	7 YEARS	CHEMICAL ENGINEER
FRANCISCO SÁ	26 YEARS	IDEM	11 MONTHS	SECRETARY/RESEARCH ASSISTANT
IVAN PESSOA	47 YEARS	43 YEARS	4 YEARS	MECHANICAL ENGINEER
LUIZ CLÁUDIO	36 YEARS	35 YEARS	1 YEAR	COMPANY ADMINISTRATOR

SUBJECT	OCCUPANCY	INCOME PERSON	INCOME FAMILY	RESIDENCE
MILTON	PUBLIC SERVANT	MORE THAN	R$ 6.500	SÃO JOSÉ DO RIO
GARDEN	FEDERAL	R$ 4,000		BLACK
TOMÁZLINS	SCHOOL DRIVER	R$ 4.500	-	GARDEN

EDÚJOSÉ	ENGINEER	R$ 4.000	-	PAULISTA GREAT BEACH
FRANCISCO SA	CONSULTANT SECRETARY / *JIU-JITSU* TEACHER	R$ 2.500 R$2000 + 500	IDEM. WIFE NO WORK	BUTANTÃ
IVAN PESSOA	BUSINESS	R$ 2.700		ALTO DA LAPA
LUIZ CLÁUDIO	ADMINISTRATOR COMPANIES	R$ 2.300	R$ 7.000	INTERLAGES

SUBJECT	STATE CIVIL	F S ISLAND	RELIGION	"RACE"
MILTON GARDEN	MARRIED	NO	CATHOLIC	WHITE
TOMÁZ LINS	SINGLE	NO	EVANGELICAL	WHITE
EDÚ JOSÉ	SINGLE	NO	ATHEIST	WHITE
FRANCIS-CO SA	MARRIED	NO	ATHEIST	BROWN LIGHT BROWN
IVAN PESSOA	DIVORCED	YES, 3.	DOESN'T HAVE ONE, BUT BELIEVES IN GOD.	WHITE
LUIZ CLÁUDIO	SINGLE	NO	ECLECTIC CATHOLIC	BLACK NOT LEGITIMATE BROWN

5.4.2 . Category analysis: motivation for semen donation

The aim of this study was to investigate sperm donation in order to find out the factors governing the motivation of men who register with semen banks to provide their reproductive cells free of charge and under the rule of anonymity. The results will be analysed in the light of the theory of the gift, pioneered by Mareei Mauss.

According to the data collected at the field study stage, where six people who regularly donate sperm were interviewed in person, it was found that semen donation falls within the sphere of gift-giving.

The reasons that led these men to become sperm donors were not entirely rational. As presented in section 5.3.2, the interviews conducted promoted real "encounters", which provided a favourable space for delving deeper and discovering the feelings and logic involved in the decision to provide sperm to a semen bank. In these "encounters", the testimonies made it clear how the stages of selecting subjects, which are necessary for their acceptance as donors and for maintaining this status, resulted in painful experiences for many of them, in varying senses. In order to continue with their life goal, or "mission", as Edu put it, these men had to "break down barriers", transcend limitations, re-signify values, as they travelled a path full of conflicts, most of which were related to feelings of fear and embarrassment.

The data collected in the research indicated that all the subjects donate their genetic material to a semen bank for two main reasons: to *help others* and to *perpetuate themselves.*

"Helping others" has two aspects: one direct and the other indirect. Directly, helping others represents, for the interviewees, the contribution made to men and women who wish to procreate but are prevented from doing so due to infertility problems, even if this infertility is in the social sphere, which refers to single individuals and homosexuals. The following quote exemplifies the type of "direct help to others":

> I want to see... no, I want someone else to feel the emotion I felt when I saw my son for the first time. The doctor opened the little window and showed me him: my son. So to know that someone else felt what I felt through the semen I donated. Just talking about it makes me feel so emotional!" (Ivan)

Indirectly helping people who use heterologous reproduction means that, at first level, the donation of semen is motivated by the donor's personal goals. On a second level, helping others becomes a consequence of the act of supplying sperm to the bank. In other words, the direct modality favours the recipient and the indirect modality prioritises the donor. However, both modalities - direct and indirect - are considered to be gifts because they are also used in the same types of procedures aimed at pregnancy. For example, Milton cited the following as factors that motivated him to donate: the desire to have many children, the desire to have children with ethnic variations, and the intention that the semen bank should continue to exist, so that it can help his wife, should the need arise one day. Edu, on the other hand, cited as the reasons that led him to donate: procreation as a way of "circumventing" death, and procreation as a life mission. The following statements exemplify the *indirect type of helping others.*

> I decided to donate semen in order to fulfil my goal in life, which is to reproduce. So I was thinking mainly of myself. It's not that I want to hurt people, no. It's not like that. I'm not the kind of person who wants people to get hurt. But when I made the donation, I did it with myself in mind. That's how it was, but of course they'll benefit too. (Edu)

> Can I talk about what prompted me to donate? So it was to circumvent death. I realised that procreation is the main mission of human beings, which is to be born, live, reproduce and die. (Edu)

> It was an exchange of favours. The person who wants to... the woman who wants to get pregnant and can't because the man is sterile, or one is incompatible with the other, they'll be able to have a child with my semen, which is frozen there. On the other hand, I, who like this family thing, and I don't have a way yet, I don't have a girlfriend or anything, will be able to be a father. It's a little seed of mine that's going to sprout and be looked after by someone out there." (Luiz Cláudio)

The group studied was divided as to whether they belonged to the two modes of altruism, i.e. half were more strongly involved in the direct sphere (Tomaz, Francisco and Ivan) and the other half in the indirect sphere (Milton, Edu and Luiz Cláudio). However, it was found that the agents interchange between the two ways of helping others.

Still on the subject of this type of motivation, it was interesting to note that the men who said they donated semen for personal reasons remained rooted in a self-perception geared towards selfishness or self-centredness, showing a certain difficulty with the opposite position. As the interviews developed, it was possible to observe that these individuals often behave generously in their day-to-day lives. They are often willing to listen to their loved ones when they are going through difficult times; they usually lend money, even if they don't have the amount requested; they are regular donors of other human materials, such as blood and organs; and they agreed to take part in this research in response to my request to collaborate.

The interviewees became clearer about the issue as their statements were confronted, which highlighted certain incoherencies and inconsistencies in relation to generosity/selfishness. The following quote illustrates this:

> I'd never thought about it before, I'd never realised... It's true. Even if the donor thinks of his own motives first, he's acting to help people who need it, because the semen is going to help someone who wants to have a child and can't. (Edu)

Another dimension of the motivation for donating semen is related to the *desire for perpetuation.* All of the survey participants mentioned their interest in the continuity of their existence, and that of the human species, through the descendants that will come from the material provided to the bank. This idea is based on the notion that they themselves extended the existence of their ancestors with their birth, which is a reason to thank their parents and God. In this sense, contributing to someone's conception is as much about keeping one's own life preserved when it no longer exists as it is about contributing to the perpetuity of one's ancestry. The phenomenon would occur, according to the group, through the transmission of their genetic determinants, or even through the passing on of their immaterial characteristics, such as moral values, temperament, personality and others.

Another factor mentioned by half of the interviewees as a reason for donating semen was the *desire to guarantee paternity status.* As Tomaz, Edu and Luiz Cláudio do not currently have any concrete idea of forming a family, from which their children would come, they felt motivated to donate semen as a way of guaranteeing that they will be parents one day, even if they never meet their offspring.

The same was not mentioned by the other interviewees, since the remaining three already take fatherhood for granted. Ivan already has children and the others: Milton and Francisco are married and waiting for news of their wives' pregnancies.

Motivation as a way of guaranteeing paternity *status is* consistent with the material already covered in this thesis, in section 2.1. *Social medicalisation and the desire for offspring.*

The desire to procreate seems to be a hegemonic tendency in most human societies, where there is a need to solve the problem of childlessness, both biologically and socially, implying more or less visible arrangements between individuals of both sexes, indicating at the same time that sterility has always been socially frowned upon and repudiated as an unfortunate condition. According to anthropologist Françoise Héritier, the desire for children and offspring is based on the notion that: (...) Not to transmit life is to break a chain in which no one is the ultimate end and is, on the other hand, to forbid *oneself* access to the *status of* ancestor (HÉRITIER, 2000, p. 103).

Narcissism was another motivating factor for gamete donation, and this element emerged from the interviews conducted directly and indirectly. It should be made clear here that we are not referring to the type of narcissism interpreted by psychoanalysis[31] . In this study, the expression has the meaning of self-admiration and love for oneself, rather than the excessive self-aggrandisement characteristic of Narcissus from Greek mythology, a character famous for his admiration of his own beauty.

Milton was the agent who clearly mentioned narcissism as one of the factors that motivated him to donate sperm to a semen bank. According to him, he was self-admiring both in physical and aesthetic terms, and in a moral sense. In a country where corruption, malice, theft, lies, dishonesty, disloyalty, hidden interests, among many other bad character traits, are commonplace, Milton seeks to cultivate attitudes and behaviours that are the opposite, by being frank, sincere, kind, honest, loyal, friendly and correct with the people in his personal and professional life. He also endeavours to be upright in his duties as a citizen.

Milton's life goal, based on correction and benevolence, follows a personal objective, even differing from the behaviour he observed from his parents, especially from the father figure.

As for his body, Milton sees his own image as beautiful, especially his face. With the exception of his big toe and the colour of his eyeballs, which are not so white,

[31] In psychoanalysis, the term narcissism (a) appeared for the first time in Freud in 1910, to explain the choice of object in homosexuals; they "... take themselves as a sexual object; they start from narcissism and look for young people who look like them, and whom they can love as their mother loved them" (1a). The discovery of narcissism led Freud to propose - in The Schreber Case, 1911 - the existence of a phase of sexual evolution intermediate between auto-eroticism and object love. "The subject begins by taking himself, his own body, as an object of love" (2), which allows for a first unification of sexual drives. In Totem and Taboo (1913) he expresses the same point of view. Freud had already used the concept of narcissism before "introducing" it through a special study (On Narcissism: An Introduction [Zur Einfuhrung dês Narzissmus, 1914]). But in this text, it is in the whole of psychoanalytic theory that he introduces the concept, particularly considering libidinal investments (LAPLANCHE; PONTALIS, 2001, p. 287).

he loves himself as a whole. He appreciates the moments when he is alone, in the peace and quiet of his being, when he feels as if his person is enough for him. Therefore, in his leisure time, he likes to prioritise activities that can be practised individually, such as fishing and bird breeding: his favourite *hobbies*. This

Therefore, for Milton, the act of donating semen aims to multiply his being, spreading his physical and moral gifts throughout the world.

Indirectly, the other agents showed some self-admiration and love for themselves, as well as a desire to pass on their physical and moral characteristics to their descendants. However, they didn't emphasise this vehemently, as happened with Milton.

In addition to self-contemplation, the data collected in the research pointed to the *capacity for contemplation* as another factor that led two agents to donate sperm. Here, the meaning of contemplation differs from the contemplation referred to above, constituting a knowledge of God or divinity, not through religious practice or its discursive methods, but through experiencing the divine. This phenomenon was mentioned by both Ivan and Milton. The latter said that he donates semen as a way of thanking God for everything he is as a person, and for everything that life has offered him, because he has everything: love, happiness, good financial conditions, the job he wants, and he doesn't feel like he's missing anything. According to Milton, this divine figure is infinitely greater than his own. Ivan also expressed that he feels in close contact with God and that God has already shown himself to be present, helping him in his difficulties and delivering him from intense suffering and even death. For the agent, his way of life, focused on the well-being of his neighbour, is in fact a way of pleasing God. The following quotes illustrate this:

> [The motivation for semen donation] can be gratitude for having had life [...]. Just gratitude, and enjoying life and thinking that God is much bigger than me, that he gave me everything and never lacked anything for me. (Milton)
>
> [Contact] with God? Of course. Not just contact, but I have proof that he exists through various things that have happened to me, and for me it was he who did it. He saved me, when I had the accident, I had to die, I don't know, various things. It was he who took away my father's pain three days before he died... I think so, I'm sure of it. [...] Whatever I can do, I do for others, to feel good, to serve God." (Ivan)

Another factor that has motivated some men to donate semen is linked to the collective imaginary *of users of conceptive reproductive technologies as wealthy people.* Luiz Cláudio and Tomaz idealise that the children they will have through the sperm they have provided to the bank, because they will be born through assisted reproduction, will belong to families from high social strata and that, for this reason, they will be well brought up. The quotes below illustrate the point:

> [...] And another thing... to have an insemination, not just anyone can do it, you have to be in a financially secure position to have treatment, to pay for it, because it's not cheap, so I know that I didn't put my child there... in the care of just anyone. The person has the conditions, went there, paid for it, did it and is there looking after a little seed of mine." (Tomaz)

> [...] even more so since there's been this whole process, knowing that a child has gone to a family that can provide, I don't know... I know it's for the long term, right? A good education for your child, everything else, maybe even better than you could give them yourself, or if you're lucky enough to have a father, a mother who are very good [...] But knowing that, in your mind, you're going to be with someone who can afford it, because I think most people who go for this kind of treatment are people who have a certain standard of living that's different from others, because these tests aren't cheap, right? But I believe... I think it's even better than people who adopt children from orphanages and so on, because it's a very expensive treatment. (Luiz Cláudio)

It cannot be said that all users of conceptive technology treatments are as financially well-off as Tomaz and Luiz Cláudio imagine. It is up to scientific research to expand knowledge about this phenomenon. However, the reports point to three issues. Firstly, it is clear that they both want their "children" to receive the best in terms of care and education. Secondly, the interviewees' explanations highlight a theme that has been the subject of debate in the arena of conceptive reproductive technologies: *stratified* reproduction, from which we emphasise a point raised by Brazilian and foreign researchers, arguing that CRTs are corroborating to constitute distinct classes of users: those who can and those who cannot access assisted reproductive treatments.

American feminists Ginsburg and Rapp (1995) have dedicated themselves to studies that favour a deeper understanding of the paradoxical association between consumption and motherhood in their discussion of stratified reproduction. In their book *Conceiving the new world order: the global politics of reproduction*, the authors address the issue. According to them:

> We use the term stratified reproduction [...] to describe the power relations by which some categories of people are empowered to nurture and reproduce, while others are not (GINSBURG; RAPP, 1995 apud ALLEBRANDT, 2008, p. 19).

Brazilian researcher Rosana Barbosa investigated reproductive rights in the context of CRTs, with the target audience being women who use public health services to treat infertility. According to the results obtained by Barbosa (2003), the fact that assisted reproduction results in high costs involving procedures and medicines, combined with structural aspects, contributes to the restriction of users belonging to social classes with low purchasing power, both in the public service and, above all, in the services offered by private institutions. The following quote elucidates the above:

> The new conceptive reproductive technologies have as their main clientele members of social groups with greater purchasing power, who are able to afford their high costs. Public services for the treatment of infertility, generally linked to public universities, represent the only alternative for other social groups to seek pregnancy. Many of these services don't offer all the assisted reproduction techniques and users have to pay for the medicines needed for the procedures, which restricts access, as well as having a long waiting list for the procedures. It's worth emphasising that there are structural aspects that hinder the existence and expansion of these services. Some are of a legal and ethical nature, such as responsibility for the conservation and safekeeping of genetic material or even the very existence of these services in the public sphere, due to the difficulties still present in access and quality of care for women's comprehensive health. (BARBOSA, 2003, p. 45).

As well as mentioning the issue of *stratified reproduction* in the context of TRCs, semen donors Luiz Cláudio and Tomaz Lins reveal another aspect of the practice of semen donation: the association between donation and adoption, referring to the third issue that emerged from the subjects' presentations.

Gamete donation is an element that is often compared to adoption, but the focus of discussions has generally been on maintaining or dissolving the anonymity of donors. In the US, there is a long-standing and well-established movement aimed at valuing the right of adopted children to know their origins. With regard to gamete donation, questions revolve around the extension of this right to the children of donors. According to the quote below:

> [...] in recent years, donor offspring have begun to ask whether they, like adoptees, have the right to information about their biological origin. Fuelled by renewed faith in the importance of genes and the victories of open adoption[32] , the so-called donor disclosure movement is prompting sperm banks across the country to change the way they donate. (THE NEW *York Times-,* the year in ideas: A to Z*; OPEN sperm donation,* 09/12/2001 apud ALLEBRANDT, 2008, p. 68).

In Brazil, adoption is of a closed nature, resulting in the extraction of the biological parents' data from the adopted child's birth certificate, with only the identifying data of the adoptive parents remaining.

However, the interviewees in this research addressed another aspect of the

[32] This is the type of adoption in which the birth parents' details are not deleted from the birth certificate.

association between donation and adoption. For the interviewees, donating semen also means transferring all the responsibilities involved in raising the child born from the donated sperm to the recipient, the biological mother and/or the social father, supposedly people from higher strata. In this sense, in theory, because their genetic child will belong to a class of people with greater purchasing power, a high level of education, even better than they could offer, will be guaranteed. It's worth emphasising that both interviewees revealed a personal inability to exercise paternity at the moment.

Another important aspect of the theme of the involvement of semen donation with the "money" factor that emerged from the data collected in the field study refers to the concern about future charges from the recipients and from the child generated by the donation, in relation to the donor. Tomaz explains that he experiences fears about this issue, as can be seen in the following quote:

> I was really worried that someone would take my details and then turn up at the house saying that I have a child and that I have to pay maintenance. Can you imagine? I was worried about that, but then I thought about the seriousness of the clinic and that shouldn't happen. If it does, I can prove that I made the donation and it won't cost me anything." (Tomaz)

Edu José doesn't experience the same feelings as Tomaz, but he reveals that he is often warned by those close to him about the possibility of being questioned in the future by the children born from his semen, who could claim money or inheritance. Let's look at the following quote:

> [...] because a lot of people say: 'Oh, the guys will take your money later, they'll want an inheritance, I don't know what...' But, yeah... I also think that, if that's the case... I think that what we bring to life isn't so much the money, it's not so much what we bring... it's the question of sensitivity, of having a child, of the guy knowing that I'm his father, that he's my son. I think that's much more important than *the* question of money. If he's an *arsehole* and steals my money, fine, I won't take it up... (Edu José)

The aim of this work is to discuss the motivation for semen donation, based on the theory of the gift, mainly on the theorists Mareei Mauss and Jacques Godbout, whose reflections served as a foundation for the objectives of the thesis, as presented in chapter 3.

According to Mauss' analyses, the spheres of the state and the market, which are constant in modern societies, are not universal, but interpersonal systems of reciprocity can be found in all societies, from which the theorist proposed that social life is constituted by a constant give and take, based on a tension between obligation and spontaneity in the world of exchange. The leitmotif *of the Essay on the Gift* is the notion of "alliance", in which various aspects of the gift are implicated.

Another analysis by the sociologist on the subject of reciprocity as a basis for solidarity alludes to three moments in the phenomenon: *giving, receiving and giving back,* based on which the good donated would have a symbolic function that would oblige retribution, favouring the creation of social ties.

Furthermore, Mauss elaborates a dialectic regarding the gift: every exchange presupposes some kind of alienability, because when you give, you always give something of yourself; when you accept, the recipient accepts something from the giver. In this way, the subject ceases to be an independent other, albeit momentarily, because "giving and receiving" implies not only a material exchange, but also a spiritual exchange, a communication between souls, whose dimension is much broader than the utilitarian view of the gift.

It should be emphasised that the gift referred to here does not have the content that common sense attributes to the word, of charity and blessing, reducing the gift to a religious phenomenon. In the theory of the gift, there is *an organisational logic of the social that has a universalising character, in which the gift appears as a moral rule that is imposed on the community.* The aim of this study was to extend Mauss' theoretical contribution, which focused on "primitive" societies, creating interfaces with contemporary studies on the subject, which prioritise the humanisation of social relations.

Based on the data collected in the field study, it can be said that semen donation in the Brazilian context falls within the sphere of the gift. In the interviews, it was found that most of the group approached the practice driven by voluntarism, and that all of the actors feel motivated to the act by altruistic reasons, represented by the desire to help others, either directly or indirectly. More precisely, by providing healthy gametes, the agents are trying to help those individuals who want to procreate but are unable to due to their infertile status. Furthermore, within this society, the act is carried out free of charge and in favour of unknown subjects.

Added to these factors, with greater frequency, is the desire to perpetuate oneself and humanity, and the intention to guarantee the *status of* paternity. To a lesser extent, data was collected on: narcissism, characterised by self-admiration and the desire to distribute oneself in terms of uprightness of character and physical beauty; the desire for their offspring to receive a high-level education, to be provided by recipients who would belong to high socio-economic strata, in the imagination of two subjects. To them, the donors would transfer the responsibilities that the interviewees felt incapable of taking on. In addition, the ability to contemplate the deity, to whom gratitude and services are owed, was mentioned.

I propose thinking about the phenomenon of semen donation from two perspectives: one micro and one macro. The micro view of donation refers to the interaction between the main social actors, who are the donor and the recipient. The macro view covers the whole system of semen donation, encompassing medical institutions specialising in HT and semen banks, as well as the two other actors.

Focusing on the main actors: the donor, who provides the gametes, and the recipient, who receives the material and initiates the process of generating the offspring, "the constant presence of a system of interpersonal reciprocities is observed, which participates in human life and is relevant to the production of society", from which some characteristics of the gift can be highlighted. Firstly, through the act itself of providing gametes free of charge to the creators of reproduction, the gifts of *sharing* and *generosity* are generated.

Secondly, there is the establishment of the "alliance" between the parties, which is the leitmotif of Mauss' gift theory. The donor/recipient bond is established on the basis of a common goal: to generate a descendant (gift of *filiation* and gift of *family),* for which the donor gives their reproductive cells to the recipient who receives them, fertilises them, develops them (consanguineous alliance), gives birth to them (gift of *life)* and offers them the appropriate care (gift of *generosity*), through which another type of alliance is established: the descendant will give life back to the donor and the recipient, guaranteeing the continuity of the dyad, while at the same time giving it the *status of* ancestry.

Thirdly, involving the paradox of the gift, the material donated transmits to the other the material and immaterial characteristics of the donor (transmission of things and souls), which can be ambiguous. They can include beauty, uprightness of character, benevolence and sincerity (gifts in themselves), as well as the non-beautiful, capacities for evil and lying, or even physical and psychological pathologies (poison-gifts). This aspect contains the notion of *hau* (the spirit of the thing), from which there is an exchange between souls, or a spiritual exchange, which has a much broader dimension than the utilitarian view of the gift.

Therefore, we can think of the link between the recipient and the donor, which includes the child they have given birth to, through the prism of the *hau.* Through the triad, a type of bond and an exchange of souls can be formed that will go beyond anonymity, spanning generations. Inevitably, one will be imprinted on the trajectory of the other. The donor, when thinking about their child, their appearance, their way of being, the legacies they will carry from their anonymous father. The recipient, by observing a phenotypical feature in the child that differs from the biological mother, such as the shape of the fingers, for example. Also, by identifying a trait that is equivalent to the donor's data, but diverges from the characteristics of the recipient couple (or woman). An example might be the fact that the offspring has musical inclinations in a family that doesn't, while the semen donor is listed as a conductor under "profession" in the semen bank's list of donors.

Based on an understanding of society in which there is a close link between its symbolic dimension and the obligation to give, receive and reciprocate, we can cite the following as the triad of semen donation, at the very least: the act of donating semen (giving) - the use of the material by the recipient (receiving) - the birth of the baby through the recipient (reciprocating) - the return of the donor for another donation (giving/returning), and so on.

Thinking of semen donation in the light of the idea of the circulation of gifts and counter-gifts, corresponding to a *total social fact,* the phenomenon would encompass various domains of collective life. In other words, even when we emphasise the generosity aspect of the form of exchange in question, it still implies, at the same time, a religious aspect (God as creator), an economic aspect (circulation of currency via the recipient/sperm bank, and the recipient/medical institution), a legal aspect (drafting of laws for TRCs), a political aspect (definition of these norms by the Legislative Branch), an aesthetic aspect (selection of the donor), and also the reorganisation of kinship, among others.

The theory of the gift analyses the notion of human motivations as paradoxical, governing a set of apparently free and gratuitous services, but which are obligatory and self-interested. In these terms, according to Mauss, the act of *giving is not a disinterested act, in other words, there is no such thing as a gift without the expectation of retribution*, and the fact extends to the community. With regard to the subject of this study, the expectation of retribution for semen donation can be seen based on some of the factors that govern the intention of the act, such as: the desire for self-perpetuation; the guarantee of paternity *status*; the sense of "adoption" in semen donation, from which the recipients would be seen as potential educators.

Broadening the focus to the interaction between all the actors in the phenomenon of semen donation, which would represent a network of gifts, according to the material presented in Chapter 4, we can draw on the analyses of Jacques Godbout, who has dedicated his studies to the modern gift.

According to the author, organ and blood donations are part of a mixed gift system, rather than a pure gift system, based on the characteristics of these donations (GODBOUT, 1999, p. 107). The same terms can be extended to gamete donation, because in a mixed gift system: there is the importance of intermediaries (technical and professional) between the donor and the recipient, and of a particularly sophisticated technical-professional apparatus. These intermediaries (semen banks and clinics/hospitals specialising in ART) are not governed by the gift, but by the wage relationship. Furthermore, the technical-professional apparatus involved in the procedures in question is instrumental and ensures the transmission of the gift, and society does not accept the sale of donated "goods".

Returning to the object of study of this research, and based on the discussion of the results found, it was found that men's motivation for semen donation is governed by the gift, from which we oppose the attributions of differentiation between the two types of gamete donation: female and male, which only locate egg donation in the realm of full altruism. This rhetoric is common in the bibliography dedicated to reflections on the subject, which is usually based on notions of sexual, reproductive and gender hierarchies, whose social structures are historical and which reinforce the discrimination between men and women, as presented in subsection 2.3.

The notions of feminine and masculine, as well as the ways in which one and the other are linked to reproduction and the family, have come to associate woman and man, respectively, with dyads: passive/active, generosity/selfishness, selflessness/individualism, absence of sexuality/doubtful sexual conduct, medicalisation/masturbation, caring for offspring/supporting the family, home/work, and so on, from which, semen donation came to be related sometimes to altruism, but mostly also to pecuniary gain and transgressive behaviour.

The research showed that the field of semen donation is arduous and full of conflict-generating situations, which trigger feelings of various kinds, such as shame, fear, doubt, mistrust, loneliness, among others. What's more, the type of work they do often subjects them to criticism and fear, which comes from social interaction. On the other hand, when they come into contact with donation, they seem to go through experiences that favour the introjection of stigmatising roles, placing them in the position of "wankers", mere sperm donors, or even "breeding bulls". In these terms, the practice of donating semen would be more like carrying out a sentence than a practice that produces pleasure. Referring back to Edu's statement: "(...) people think that we come here thinking..'Oh, the guy's a wanker, I don't know

what...', but that's not it, it's the way to get it out. If I had to do something with that intention, I'd do it at home, you know?". If men had reproductive organs similar to those of women and needed surgical intercourse to donate gametes, wouldn't they also undergo the procedure?

On the other hand, the constant associations between the field of conceptive reproductive technologies and utilitarianism, which, as the term itself indicates, works in favour of procreation, may be governed by an even broader social phenomenon. Following Godbout's analyses, the modern individual is "suspicious" of gift-giving attitudes, as a result of which the gift is usually socially concealed.

His reflections on the subject are richly developed in the aforementioned book, The *Spirit of the Gift.* The text on the back cover elucidates his main thesis, which is the gift among the moderns, according to the following quote:

> Does the gift exist [still]? Modern man accepts being accused of many things, but certainly not of being naive. He could even be anything but. He knows very well what lies behind the stories of the gods, behind the myths, behind all the beautiful and great tales from all countries and all times. Modern man is a realist. He therefore knows what lies behind the gift. Having the sad but modern privilege of looking reality in the face and not letting himself be deceived by false appearances, he knows very well that what motivates the production and exchange of goods is not altruism or generosity, but material interest; that politics is not a question of ideals but of power and violence, and that affections are not commanded by feelings, but fundamentally by sex. (GODBOUT, 1999, back cover).

According to the author, modern people usually deal with the gift by denying it, or understanding it as a kind of pretence, a simulation of gratuitousness and disinterest in an environment where only interest and equivalence prevail everywhere. However, this contemporary refusal to believe in the existence of the gift seems to be an indication of a way of representing the phenomenon in an inverted way, in relation to selfish material interest. In contrast, the "true" gift can only be gratuitous. Since gratuitousness is impossible, the true gift is conceived as equally impossible. Paradoxically, the denial of the gratuitousness of human motivations attests to the reality of their gift. For, according to the author: "we need to think of the gift not as a series of unilateral and discontinuous acts, but as a relationship, and there is no such thing as a one-way, gratuitous and meaningless relationship" (GODBOUT, 1999, p. 16).

> Even more than capital, according to Marx, the gift is not a thing, but a social relationship. It is even the social relationship par excellence, a relationship that is more fearsome than one would like. The idea that the gift is always self-

> interested and the idea that it should always be free have in common the fact that they give an aseptic view of the gift, as well as preventing us from realising that if it is conjured up and denied by the moderns to such an extent, it is because it is dangerous. (GODBOUT, 1999, p. 16).

The utilitarian point of view that dominates today has led Western man to believe that he must always win. And as if debts, even insignificant ones, are intrinsically dangerous and unbearable, unless you feel a certain pleasure in giving something back. In this sense, "in the face of the risks inherent in any gift, money and recourse to a mercantilist logic are the antidotes - both counter-donations and counter-poisons - par excellence." (GODBOUT, 1999, p. 17). The idea is justified by the notion that in the market system, things only have value between themselves, whereas in the gift system, things are worth in terms of what the relationship is worth, and this is fuelled by what circulates between people. Thus, selfishness seems to be more of a response to a

solidarity that has been imposed on the recipient, and which they don't want, since the way not to feed the unwanted gift is to remain in the market sphere.

Based on Godbout's analyses, the social sciences have accustomed us to interpreting history and the social game as products of the strategies of rational agents who seek to maximise the satisfaction of their material interests, which is the dominant "utilitarian" view. In order to see the gift, whether in everyday life or in academia, we will have to deconstruct the vision of the gift as love, that sung love, that love of poetry.

On the other hand, it (the gift) does not resemble its religious representation, especially since the Reformation, when people have come to believe that only God can truly grant his grace freely, be benevolent and generous, something that is denied to the exteriority of transcendence.

In addition, it will be necessary to break with the variants of *Nietzscheanism*, which present the human being as a natural egoist, and with its modern Western variant, which represents man as a power-hungry being.

According to the author, there is no doubt that the modern individual is constantly involved in gift relationships, but the modern gift represents an original form of circulation that is different from the one studied by Mauss and most of the authors who study the subject and who reject gratuitousness. There are many differences between the gift and the commercial return: *there isn't always a return* - conversely, the *return is often greater than the gift -, the return happens, even if it wasn't desired -,* in the gratuitousness that it gives rise to - recognition -, this supplement that circulates and isn't included in the account are important returns for the giver. Finally, *the return is often in the gift itself,* in the artist's inspiration, and in the personal transformation undergone by those who give, because they become greater (GODBOUT, 1999, p. 113-115).

There is a relationship between the donor, the recipient and the child generated, and a type of relationship that overcomes anonymity and will last through the ages. Furthermore, the interviews conducted indicate that the act of providing semen in favour of infertile people who want to have children neither brings a financial return, nor the return that could come from the relationship with the child born; conversely, the return happens, even if it wasn't desired; often it is greater than the gift; often the return is in the gift itself.

Let's hear it for the donors:

> For me, if I've done good for someone, if I've made someone happy, that's what matters. Living like this is good for me. (Tomaz Lins)
> I want to see... no, I want someone else to feel the emotion I felt when I saw my son for the first time. The doctor opened the little window and showed me him: my son. So to know that someone else felt what I felt through the semen I donated. Just talking about it makes me feel so emotional!" (Ivan Pessoa)

> [...] because a lot of people say: 'Oh, the guys will take your money later, they'll want an inheritance, I don't know what...' But, yeah... I also think that, if that's the case... I think that what we bring to life isn't so much the money, it's not so much what we bring... it's the question of sensitivity, of having a child, of the guy knowing that I'm his father, that he's my son. I think that's much more important than *the* question of money. If he's an *arsehole* and steals my money, fine, I won't take it up... (Edu José)

> Semen donation could be a thank you for my coming to life, but I've only just thought about it, it never entered my mind. Just thanks for enjoying life and believing that God is much bigger than me, that he has given me everything and that I have never lacked anything. Everything is my family, love, health, I have the economic condition to live well, without going through any hardship as I know many do. Life is enough for me. I don't need anything else." (Milton Jardim)

> I decided to donate semen when I saw an advert asking for donors. It was only to help people who need it, who can't have children any other way (Francisco Sá)

> Normally I'm like that... at work, even if I don't have time, I'll teach someone who's just starting out. With friends, I'm a 'jack of all trades', I'm always listening to people, to their problems, if it's money I'll lend it. I've never regretted being like that. I often say that I donate kindness. (Luiz Cláudio)

CHAPTER 6

FINAL CONSIDERATIONS

In the vast and indestructible field of assisted reproduction, this study has chosen as its object the phenomenon of semen donation in the Brazilian context. The focus of the research was on the factors that motivate men to donate sperm to a specialised bank. The results were analysed in the light of the gift theory, using the renowned scholars on the subject: *Marcel Mauss* and *Jacques Godbout* as theoretical references.

What drives men to donate semen to specialised banks? This is the question that guided this research. Through the data collected from all the subjects, some aspects stood out due to their relevance. As a result of the focus theme, important issues emerged, such as: the desire to offer help to others; the representation of son, in other words, the space that the offspring occupies in the donor's life; and finally, the prevailing sex and gender hierarchies, which would de-characterise semen donation from the sphere of gift. These issues proved to be of the utmost importance in understanding what drives a man to donate sperm in favour of infertile people, even if they are unknown and the act has no financial return.

In terms of *knowledge* about the field of reproductive technologies, and even about the world of gamete donation (eggs and sperm), all the subjects are almost lay people. The agents have a vague idea of what assisted reproduction is, limiting the field to treatments for achieving pregnancy. Even when it comes to gamete donation, the situation is similar. It turned out that the research agents have a kind of knowledge that they acquired through contact with the semen bank, through questions asked by them and to them, and through experiencing the donation process.

With regard to the regulation of the practice, the donors' knowledge is on a par with that of the field as a whole, in other words, it is practically nil. It was interesting to note that even with regard to the rules of anonymity and gratuity that directly involve gamete donation, the group had the same level of knowledge: little to none. It is worth noting that in order to comply with the terms of the regulations in question, donors usually sign a *term of commitment when* they first contact the semen bank, in which they register their agreement with the legal requirements.

One of the group's members, a legal professional, stood out. In his opinion, the CFM's resolution is fragile for dealing with situations that may arise in the future, as the anonymity rule is antagonistic to the right to recognise paternity and to know one's biological origins, which are included in the Brazilian Constitution. On the subject, the agent proposed an anonymity option: pure or conditional. "Pure anonymity" refers to the current situation. Conditional anonymity means agreeing to have one's identity exposed and maintaining contact with the receiving party (parents and children). The interviewee would opt for the second type of anonymity.

The other interviewees were divided on the subject. Two of them would choose to keep their identity anonymous. One of the agents is against anonymity. The last two interviewees also expressed an interest in bonding with the children born from their donations, but they were obedient to current regulations.

All the interviewees were in favour of the practice being free of charge, as the opposite could encourage people who don't like working to become "professional sperm donors". The group prefers not to be paid for the donation, but questions the possibility of being offered a stipend to reimburse expenses that end up being borne by the donor. In addition, in order to recognise, thank and repay the donation, the semen bank could change some of the attitudes it has towards its agents. Discrimination can be seen in the different treatment received when arriving and leaving the clinic. In the former there is attention and warmth; in the latter, loneliness. Although this seems to be an obvious behavioural strategy on the part of the semen bank, the way in which the semen donation process is completed could be modulated to suit individual expectations, and other ways of completing the act could be created. Furthermore, some men complained of a lack of privacy when visiting the semen bank and improving this condition would be a way of repaying them. Finally, other types of recognition/retribution were mentioned: the offer of snacks and gifts.

When it came to their *opinion on gamete donation,* the group was in favour, because the technique helps in cases of infertility. For two subjects, the subject should be more widely disseminated in the mass media, where stories and programmes are based more on real facts and less on fiction, which is often far removed from reality. This would make it possible to dispel both the misinformation and the distortions and ironies that usually permeate the subject.

Another complained about the lack of psychological services for all those involved in artificial reproduction, whether it was to promote assessment, guidance or to offer psychological support to individuals. Finally, one of the donors limited himself to supporting choices. He cares about his choice at the moment: to donate semen.

With regard to the decision to reveal or conceal one's status as a semen donor from social relationships, it was found that the group's attitude was governed by a variety of factors, such as: the type of personality of the social actor; the rigidity or openness of the environment to which the agent belongs with regard to behaviour "outside the norms" of society; the meaning that the donation has in their life, which would be linked to the motivation for the practice.

Of the total, only one agent keeps the donation completely separate from his social environment. This situation seems to be due to a number of factors: the degree of importance that the act had for his life: responding to a request from an advert recruiting candidates to be sperm donors; the personality of the interviewee, who is more rational than emotional. As such, the value attributed to sperm donation would be confined to his initial objective, and should not belong to the other sectors of his life. Another factor that seems to reinforce the subject's position is the fact that his family (wife and parents) are very strict about anything that deviates from "normal", a fact that gives him the certainty that his family will reject his attitude.

As for the rest of the group, all the men who told or would tell their loved ones about their experience showed themselves to be flexible, for the most part, and also to have a great deal of autonomy in terms of their choices and attitudes. Three agents revealed themselves as sperm donors to people close to them, and the fact that there had been and still is criticism or agreement never influenced their decision, precisely because, as well as being determined, semen donation represents a life "mission". For this reason, they attribute inestimable value to the act.

One of the interviewees fits the profile of the group above. However, he keeps the matter secret, solely because he is complying with what was requested by the semen bank: that he keep his status as a donor anonymous. The agent said that his stance on the matter is the result of the importance he attaches to his word, as proof of enforcing an agreement made informally between the parties. However, his preference would be to be able to share with everyone the joy he feels at donating semen.

As far as the last actor is concerned, he first chose to carry out a type of "opinion poll" in his social environment, with the intention of finding out his interlocutors' responses on the subject. The interviewee revealed the experience he had had, but indirectly, in other words, another protagonist was used to represent the semen donor in the story he told his closest family and friends. As the vast majority reacted negatively, with only one friend giving a favourable opinion, the donor decided to keep his experience hidden.

With regard to semen users, most of the actors were in favour of anyone using their gametes. However, two actors were resistant to homosexuals. The reasons they gave were equivalent and were based on the naturalised idea of marriage, reproduction, family and kinship based on heterosexism. Thus, for both interviewees, people who have affective and erotic relationships with the same sex are seen as deviant, "affected", outside "normal" biological and social standards. In addition, the refusal of the two donors became even more intense when they thought of their own "children" being cared for and educated by two mums or dads, which could lead to significant maladjustments in the children. In this sense, based on their position, homosexuals would be excluded as recipients, an opinion that was softened when we thought about the atrocities that tend to inhabit our daily lives, whether we experience them ourselves or through the news.

As for the *donor as recipient* item, which investigated acceptance of the use of donated semen, the group was divided. Half were in favour of using gametes cryopreserved in a specialised clinic. Of the other half, two were preliminarily opposed, with infertility treatment as their first option. In the event of failure, both would opt for adoption, as they would not be the children's biological parents, and the act of adoption seems more humane than ART. However, for the agents, receiving semen from anonymous donors could be made possible in an attempt to fulfil their wives' wishes. The sixth subject remained neutral. The choice of whether or not to use the semen bank would depend on the occasion and, above all, on what was best for his wife.

With the items *destination of the donated semen, representation of a child,* and *idealisation of the child resulting from the donation,* the aim was to find out how the agents deal with the anonymous sphere of semen donation, which takes shape immediately after their reproductive cells have been given to the bank. In general, the group showed that they were not fixated on the events after the sperm was collected. Firstly, as the agents have very limited knowledge of the field, including the details of the donated material's journey (laboratory, semen culture, freezing, registration, contacting the specialist and/or the recipient, payment and proof of the act, delivery of the canister with the inseminating dose, receiving the container from the clinic or hospital, preparing the patient for insemination, scheduling the procedure, treating the semen, carrying out the insemination, pregnancy [if successful], gestation and birth of the baby), there is a difficulty in making an imaginary control of the destination of the semen. So when some people think about it, they tend to focus on: the nobility of the cause, the concern felt about possible illegalities that could occur with the cells, the circulation of the gametes, and the "child".

As for the supposed descendants, the group was divided between satisfaction and concern. Two agents expressed concern about the type of education being given to the children, whether they were being treated well or, conversely, if they were being mistreated. In addition, both individuals expressed a desire to take part in the lives of these "children" as "parents", giving advice on any doubts they might have, taking part in leisure time and having fun, and providing financial support if necessary. It's worth pointing out that, when talking about their "children" as "parents", the interviewees expressed a certain withdrawal, as if they had no right to their wishes.

The feeling of satisfaction related to biological children is based on the imagination of two actors, who associate the users of conceptive technologies with higher social strata. In this sense, their children would be receiving a higher level of education than their financial circumstances would allow them to offer.

The results obtained point to the fact that the messages emitted by these four agents draw on the characteristics attributed to the model of fatherhood that circulates in our society, to which could be added the concern that some of the interviewees expressed about the idea that the recipients and main carers of "their children" might turn out to be homosexual individuals, as mentioned above. In addition to these four, another interviewee said that he attributed to himself a kind of "father" role in relation to the "child" he thought existed, but in this case paternity would be limited to affection. For his part, he would like to meet the child, introduce them to his children who, in his view, would have them as a sister and, even if anonymously, he only wishes them well and that they are a good person, just like the children he has brought up.

Finally, for one of the agents, the child born from his semen does not occupy the position of "his child", because the subject represents filiation based on the bonds established through living together within the family.

The whole group represents offspring as continuity and as part of itself. Like a seed that is born, lives, germinates, produces new seeds and dies, the agents will be reborn through their children, and so on. According to the donors, the transmission of biological and subjective characteristics is the result of both genetic factors and the social construction of the subject. Two of the interviewees attributed greater value to learning in the social environment, compared to the genetic load.

Most of them long for the experience of fatherhood, and only one of them has children. Two agents are on the verge of realising this ideal, two others are waiting for this moment, but don't even have a commitment to a woman, and one of the interviewees doesn't intend to procreate for two main reasons: because of personal and financial incapacity, in terms of care and expenses, and because he can't conceive of the idea of a child coming from him to be part of a world that, in his view, is quite chaotic.

As far as semen donation itself is concerned, most of the agents became involved with the phenomenon voluntarily. Five of them were moved to the practice by a personal desire, in some cases without a plausible explanation. One person decided to donate in response to a newspaper advert for a semen bank.

All the semen donors presented themselves as people who cultivate the virtue of generosity as a way of life. As well as gametes, they are donors of other types of human material, such as blood, organs and bone marrow. They often donate/loan their possessions to those in need (clothes, shoes, money). Their character is upright, sincere, obliging, fair and benevolent. The very interest of the vast majority of the group in taking part in the research was driven by the desire to contribute. This being the case, and in conjunction with all the research data, it can be said that semen donation was motivated by altruistic issues, since the main reason for providing gametes to a semen bank is the desire to help an infertile individual who wants a child.

In addition to the desire to help others, the other factors identified as governing semen donation were: the desire to perpetuate; the intention to guarantee the *status* of father; the existence of a narcissism based on self-admiration, from which there would be a desire to transmit oneself as a gift to the world; the intention that the "child" would receive high-level care; and, finally, the ability to contemplate the divine, both as a form of gratitude for the gift of life and as a desire to serve God.

The accounts of some of the agents about the experience of semen donation, especially during the first contacts, reinforced the concept of the phenomenon as a gift, as they showed that the field of this type of donation is arduous, even painful, and crossed by countless conflicts that had to be overcome in order to achieve the goal. Because sperm collection requires masturbation, the practice is usually surrounded by taboos and fantasies that often turn the gift into a stigma, embarrassment, doubt and loneliness. This reality was observed as a "fog", or a "climate" that surrounds visits to the semen bank: in the glances in the building's foyer; in the difference in treatment given to sperm donors on entering and leaving the clinic; in the conflicts that arise from contact with a laboratory next to the collection room: its technological apparatus and its staff; in the need to hide the condition of semen donor from the social environment.

Sperm donation also belongs to the sphere of the gift, if we change the lens to the theory of the gift, because the practice provides fulfilment of Mauss' triple obligation of giving/receiving/retributing in the following stages: supply of the sperm/use of the material by the recipient/treatment and pregnancy/new donation.

Analysing the phenomenon of heterologous reproduction as a *total social fact,* by highlighting the generosity aspect of semen donation, it still implies, at the same time, a religious aspect (God as creator), an economic aspect (circulation of currency via the semen recipient/bank, and the recipient/medical institution), a legal aspect (drafting of laws for CRTs), a political aspect (definition of these rules by the Legislative Branch), an aesthetic aspect (selection of the donor), and also the reorganisation of kinship, among others.

In terms of the paradox of gratuitousness and obligation in semen donation, the expectation of retribution can be seen in certain factors motivating the act, such as: the desire for self-perpetuation; the guarantee of paternity *status*; and the sense of "adoption" in semen donation. By encompassing all the agents, semen donation would belong to a mixed gift system.

It's interesting to note that, in addition to generosity, semen donation is often linked to pecuniary gain, selfishness and deviant behaviour. Contemporary gift theory may be one of the justifications for this, as it elucidates that in modernity the gift is denied and limited to pretence and utilitarianism. This would occur due to an inversion in the way the phenomenon is represented, placing it as necessarily gratuitous, whereas it is necessary to think of the gift as a relationship, which does not exist as gratuitous, as unilateral and meaningless. The following facts also make up the phenomenon of mistrust towards the modern gift: the view of the gift as something from the sphere of poetry and the romantic; the variants of *Nietzscheanism,* which present the human being as a natural egoist, and with its modern Western variant, which represents man as a power-hungry being; the belief that only God can truly grant his grace freely, be benevolent and generous; the interpretations of the social sciences about history and the social game, as products of the strategies of rational agents seeking to maximise the satisfaction of their material interests.

In addition, in the field, social constructions referring to male and female sex and gender markers have emerged as reinforcers of these "suspicions" directed at sperm donation as a gift, at the intra- and extra-subject levels. Studies on the subject have emphasised that motivations for gamete donation vary between genders, with altruism generally attributed to females and utilitarianism associated with males. On the other hand, it was found that some of the people involved in this investigation found it difficult to admit altruism for themselves, as a reflection of the roles assigned to men and women. In light of the above, we would like to point out that the results found in this research are contrary to these social constructs. On the contrary, the motivation for semen donation in the Brazilian context belongs to the sphere of gift.

Modern gift theory states that the contemporary individual is constantly involved in gift relationships, but represented by an original form of circulation that is different from that studied in the past, which was dedicated to the gift in traditional societies. There are many differences between *the* gift and the mercantile return: *there is not always a return* - conversely, *the return is often greater than the gift - the return happens, even if it was not desired:* in the gratuitousness that it gives rise to - recognition - this supplement that circulates and is not included in the account are important returns for the giver. Finally, *the return is often in the gift itself,* in the artist's inspiration, and in the personal transformation undergone by those who give, because they become greater.

Following Mareei Mauss, in my opinion, semen donation can be understood as a modern gift, because there is a relationship between the triad: donor, recipient and offspring, and it is a type of relationship that overlaps anonymity, space and time. Semen donation doesn't bring a financial return, nor does it bring the return of a face-to-face relationship with the child born. On the other hand, there is a return, even if you didn't want it. Often it is greater than the gift. Often, the return is in the gift itself.

Finally, the study suggests some questions for further research, so that understanding of the subject can be deepened. The first line of enquiry could be comparative research into Western notions of sex/gender in gamete donation. A second line of reflection and research could be developed on social stratification in semen donor selection. A third line of research could be carried out with the families that receive donated gametes, in order to find out how their members build bonds of affection, as well as how they deal with the anonymous subject of the donor of reproductive cells (semen and eggs).

REFERENCES

ABDELMASSIH, Roger. Everything for a baby. *Folha de São Paulo,* São Paulo, 9 December 1994.

ALLEBRANDT, Débora. *Covering up origins, discovering relationships',* a comparative analysis of the anonymity of gamete donors in assisted reproduction. 2008. 119p. Dissertation (Master's) - Institute of Philosophy and Human Sciences, Federal University of Rio Grande do Sul, Porto Alegre, 2008.

. Between movement and interdiction: new conceptive reproductive technologies being put into practice. In: ALLEBRANDT, Débora; MACEDO, Juliana Lopes de (Org.). *Fabricating life',* ethical, cultural and social implications of the use of new reproductive technologies. Porto Alegre: Metrópole, 2007. p. 127-143.

. Family, donor anonymity and adoption: dialogues and conceptions. In: MACEDO,

Juliana Lopes de (Org.) *Fabricating life* - ethical, cultural and social implications of the use of new reproductive technologies. Porto Alegre: Metrópole, 2007. p. 67-79.

.; MACEDO, Juliana Lopes de. Paths travelled: access to NRTCT and its implications. In:*F* MACEDO, Juliana Lopes de (Org.) *Fabricating life* - ethical, cultural and social implications of the use of new reproductive technologies. Porto Alegre: Metrópole, 2007. p. 11-25.

APPIAH, Kwame Anthony. *In my father's house* Africa in the philosophy of culture. Rio de Janeiro: Contraponto, p. 273, 1997.

ARAGÃO, Luiz Tarlei. In the name of the mother: structural position and social dispositions surrounding the category of mother in Mediterranean civilisation and Brazilian society.
PERSPECTIVAS antropológicas da mulher 3. Rio de Janeiro: Zahar, 1983.

ARAÚJO, Joel Zito. The denial of Brazilian racial diversity. *Perspectives on Health and Reproductive Rights,* n. 4, year 2, p. 72, 2001.

ARKSEY, Hilary. Expert and lay participation in the construction of medicai knowledge.
Sociology of health and illness, N. 16, n. 4, p. 448-468, 1994.

BARBOSA, Rosana. New conceptive reproductive technologies: producing different classes of women? In: GROSSI, Miriam; PORTO, Rozeli; TAMANINI, Marlene (Org.). *Novas tecnologias reprodutivas conceptivas',* questões e desafios. Brasília: Letras Livres, 2003. 196p.

BARDIN, Laurence. *Content analysis.* Lisbon: Edições 70, 1970.

BORLOT, Ana Maria Monteiro; TRINDADE, Zeidi Araújo. Assisted reproduction technologies and the social representations of biological children. *Estudos de Psicologia,* Natal, v. 9, n. l,p. 63-70, 2004.

BORRILLO, Daniel. The homosexual individual, the same-sex couple and homoparental families: an analysis of the French legal reality in the international context. In: LOYOLA, Maria Andréa (Org.). *Bioethics-.* reproduction and gender in contemporary society. Rio de Janeiro: ABEP; Brasília: Letras Livres, 2005. p. 175-211.

BOURDIEU, Pierre. *Outline of a theory of practice.* Lisbon: Celta, 2002. p. 227-257.

BUTLER, Judith. *Gender problems:* feminism and the subversion of identity. Rio de Janeiro: Civilização Brasileira, 2003a.

CABRAL, João de Pina. *Anthropologia da família:* apêndice IV do relatório de atividades *da* Universidade de Lisboa - Instituto de Ciências Sociais. Lisbon: UL, 2005. p. 42-68.

CAILLÉ, Alain. *Anthropology of the gift.* Rio de Janeiro: Vozes, 2000.

. Neither holism nor methodological individualism: Mareei Mauss and the paradigm of the gift. *Revista Brasileira de Ciências Sociais,* São Paulo, v. 13, n. 38, p. 5-38, 1998.

CAMARGO, Juliana Frozel de. *Human reproduction:* ethics and law. Campinas: Edicamp, 2003.

CAMPBELL, Mary. *Biochemistry.* Rio de Janeiro: Artmed, 2001.

CÂNDIDO, Antonio. *The partners of Rio Bonito.* São Paulo: Livraria Duas Cidades, 1987.

CARDOSO, Ruth. Adventures of anthropologists in the field or how to escape the pitfalls of method. *A aventura antropológica teoria e pesquisa.* CARDOSO, Ruth (Org.). São Paulo: Paz e terra antropologia, 1986. p. 95-105.

CARSTEN, Janet. Introduction: cultures of relatedness. In: CARSTEN, J. (Ed.). *Cultures of relatedness:* ncw approaches to the study of kinship. Cambridge: Cambridge University Press, 2000.

CHAZAN, Lílian K. "Meio *kilo de gente" - production of the pleasure of seeing the construction of the foetal person mediated by ultrasound:* an ethnographic study in imaging clinics in the city of Rio de Janeiro. 2005. Thesis (PhD) - Institute of Social Medicine, Rio de Janeiro State University, Rio de Janeiro, 2005. chapters 3 and 4.

FEDERAL COUNCIL OF MEDICINE (Brazil). Resolution no. 1358/92 of 1992. Provisions on ethical standards for the use of assisted reproduction techniques. São Paulo, 1992.

CORRÊA, Marilena Villela. Reproductive medicine and the desire for children. In: GROSSI, Miriam;
PORTO, Rozeli; TAMANINI, Marlene (Org.). *Novas tecnologias reprodutivas conceptivas:* questões e desafios. Brasília: Letras Livres, 2003. p. 31-40.

. New reproductive technologies: egg donation. What could be new in this field? *Cadernos de Saúde Pública,* Rio de Janeiro, v. 16, n. 3, p. 863-870, 2000.

. *New reproductive technologies:* limits of biology or biology without limits? Rio de Janeiro: EdUERJ, 2001. 263p.

.; DINIZ, Débora. New reproductive technologies: a debate awaiting regulation. In: CARNEIRO, F.; EMERICK, M. C. (Org.). *A ética e o debate jurídico sobre o acesso e uso do genoma humano.* Rio de Janeiro: Fiocruz, 2000. p. 103-112.

.;. New reproductive technologies in Brazil: a debate awaiting regulation. *SérieAnis,* Brasília, n. 10, p. 1-5, jun. 2000.

CORRÊA, Marilena Villela; LOYOLA, Maria Andréa. New reproductive technologies: new reproductive strategies? *Physis: Revista de Saúde Coletiva*, Rio de Janeiro, v. 9, n.l, p. 1-23, 1999.

COSTA, Rosely Gomes da. Commercial aspects of gamete donation: an ethical problem. *SérieAnis,* Brasília, n. 46, p. 1-5, 2006.

. Notions of nationality and race in cases of gamete donation: some aspects of the Catalan experience. *Revista Anthropológicas*, Recife, v. 18, p. 45-58, 2007.

. What can the selection of gamete donors tell us about notions of race? *Physis: Revista de Saúde Coletiva*, Rio de Janeiro, v. 14, n.2, p. 235-255, 2004.

. Reproduction and gender: paternities, masculinities and theories of conception. *Estudos Feministas*, Florianópolis, v. 10, n. 2, p. 339-356, 2002.

. Reproductive technologies and attributions of paternity and maternity. In: GROSSI, Miriam; PORTO, Rozeli; TAMANINI, Marlene. (Org.). *Novas tecnologias reprodutivas conceptivas-*, questões e desafios. Brasília: Letras Livres, 2003. p. 69-80.

. *Reproductive technologies and notions of racialisation and ethnicity.* Paper presented at the XXVII Annual Meeting of Anpocs, Caxambu, MG, 2003. (Mimeographed).

CUSSINS, Charis. Quit sniveling, cryo-baby: we'll work out which one's your mama. In: DAVIES-FLOYD, Robbie; DUMIT, Joseph (Ed.). *Cyborg babies-.* from techno-sex to techno-tots. New York: Routledge, 1998. p. 40-67.

DANIELS, Ken; HAIMES, Erica (Ed.). *Donor insemination*: international social science perspectives. Cambridge: Cambridge University Press, 1997. 185p.

DICIONÁRIO Aurélio Online. Available at: <http://www.dicionariodoaurelio.com/dicionario.php?P=Ilusao>. Accessed on: 16 June 2008.

DINIZ, Débora. Conceptive reproductive technologies: the state of the art of the Brazilian legislative debate. *Jornal Brasileiro de Reprodução Assistida,* Ribeirão Preto, v. 7, n. 3, p. 10-19, nov./dez. 2003.

DOMINGUES, Petrônio José. Blacks with white souls? The ideology of whitening within the black community in São Paulo, 1915-1930. *Estudos Afro-Asiáticos*, Rio de Janeiro, v. 24, n. 3, p. 563-599, 2002.

DOUGLAS, Mary. *Purity and danger.* São Paulo: Perspectiva, 1966. 229p.

EDWARDS, Jeanette. Explicit connections: ethnographic enquiry in north-west England. In: EDWARDS, J. et al. *Technologies of procreation* kinship in the age of assisted conception.
2. ed. London: Routledge, 1999. p. 60-85.

ESCOSSIA, F. Black Brazil ranks 101st in quality of life. *Folha de São Paulo,* São Paulo, p. C-6, 6jan. 2002.

FAUSTO-STERLING, Anne. Dueling dualisms. *Cadernos Pagu*, Campinas, n. 17-18, p. 9-80, 2002.

FIFTH, Raymond. *Primitive economics of the New ZealandMaori.* Wellington, New Zealand: Owen, 1929. p. 25-32.

FONSECA, Claudia. Widening the circle of interlocutors: or, what a "layperson" has to do with bioethical discussions in the field of assisted reproduction. In: ALLEBRANDT, Débora; MACEDO, Juliana Lopes de (Org.) *Fabricating life* - ethical, cultural and social implications of the use of new reproductive technologies. Porto Alegre: Metrópole, 2007. Afterword. p.173- 184.

. *Paths of adoption.* 2. ed. São Paulo: Cortez, 2002. 152p.

AND The truth that gave birth to doubt: paternity and DNA. *Estudos Feministas,* Florianópolis, v. 12, n. 2, p. 13-34, May/August 2004.

. Capitu's revenge: DNA, choice and destiny in the contemporary Brazilian family. In: BRUSCHINI, Cristina; UNBEHAUM, Sandra G. (Org.). *Gênero, democracia e sociedade brasileira.* São Paulo: Carlos Chagas Foundation, 2002. p. 267-295.

FRANCO-JÚNIOR, José Gonçalves; WEHBA, Salim. I Brazilian Register on the Use of Assisted Reproduction Techniques - 1992. Reprodução, v. 9, n. 3, p. 199-202, jul-set, 1994.

FRANKLIN, Sarah. Making representations: the parliamentary debate on the Human Fertilisation and Embryology Act. In: EDWARDS, J. et al. *Technologies of procreation:* kinship in the age of assisted conception. 2. ed. London: Routledge, 1999. p. 127-169.

Macarthur Foundation. Perspectives on Health and Reproductive Rights, n. 4, year 2, 2001.

GIL, Antonio Carlos. *Methods and techniques of social research.* São Paulo: Atlas, 1999. 206p.

GINSBURG, Faye D.; RAPP, Rayna (Org.). *Conceiving the new world order.* the global politics of reproduction. Berkeley, University of California Press, 1995.

GODBOUT, Jacques T. *O espírito da dádiva.* Rio de Janeiro: Ed. Fundação Getulio Vargas, 1999. 269p.

T CAILLE, Alain. *The world of the gift.* Toronto: McGilligan Books, 2001.

GROSSI, Miriarn. Homosexual families: new families?: some reflections on gay and lesbian parenthood in Brazil and France. In: RLAL, Carmen; TONELLI, Juracy (Org.) *Genealogies of silence* - feminism and gender. Florianópolis: Ed. Mulheres, 2004a.

GROSSI, Miriarn; PORTO, Roseli; TAMANINI, Marlene (Org.). *Novas tecnologias reprodutivas conceptivas-*, questões e desafios. Brasília: Letras Livres, 2003. 196p.

GROW, Peter. Kinship as human consciousness: the case of the Piro. Revista Mana, Rio de Janeiro, v. 3, n. 2, p. 39-65, 1997.

GRUDZINSKI, Roberta Reis. The dissemination of technological alternatives and maternity projects: the scientific discourse on egg cryopreservation. In: ALLEBRANDT, Débora; MACEDO, Juliana Lopes de (Org.) *Fabricating life:* ethical, cultural and social implications of the use of new reproductive technologies. Porto Alegre: Metrópole, 2007. p. 163172.

GUILHEM, Dirce. New reproductive technologies, ethics and legislation in Brazil: a postponed debate. *Anis Series,* Brasília, n. 18, 2000.

HAIMES, Erica. Issues of gender in gamete donation. *Social Science and Medicine,* Oxford, v. 36, n.l, p. 85-93, 1993.

HASENBALG, Carlos. Between myth and fact: racism and race relations in Brazil. In: MAIO, Marcos Chor; SANTOS, Ricardo Ventura (Org.). *Raça, ciência e sociedade.* Rio de Janeiro: Fiocruz, 1996. p. 235-249.

HEILBORN, Maria Luiza. Two is pair: sociological mechanisms of conjugality and everyday life. In:. *Dois é par.* gênero e identidade sexual em contexto igualitário. Rio de Janeiro: Garamond, 2004. p. 135-165.

. Gender and the status of women: an anthropological approach. In: WOMEN and public policies. Rio de Janeiro: IBAM, 1991. p. 23-37.

HÉRITIER, Françoise. Jupiter's thigh: reflections on the new modes of procreation. *Feminist Studies,* Florianópolis, v. 8, n. 1, p. 98-114, 2000.

HERTZ, Robert. The pre-eminence of the right hand: a study in religious polarity. In: *Religião e Sociedade,* Rio de Janeiro, n. 6. p. 99-128, 1980.

HIRSCH, Eric. Negotiated limits: interviews in south-east England. In: EDWARDS, J. et al.
Technologies of procreation: kinship in the age of assisted conception. 2. ed. London: Routledge, 1999. p. 91-121.

HYDE, Lewis. *The gift:* imagination and the erotic life or property. New York: Random House, 1983. p. 102-126.

IERVOLINO, Solange Abrocesi; PELICIONI, Maria Cecília Focesi. The use of focus groups as a qualitative methodology in health promotion. *Revista da Escola de Enfermagem da USP*, São Paulo, v. 35, n. 2, p. 115-121, jun. 2001.

JASANOFF, Sheila. *Designs on nature:* Science and democracy in Europe and the United States. Princeton: Princeton University Press, 2005.

JOHNSON, Allan G. *Dicionário de sociologia-,* guia prático da linguagem sociológica. Rio de Janeiro: J. Zahar, 1997.

KONRAD, Mônica. *Nameless relations-,* anonymity, Melanesia and reproductive gift exchange between British ova donors and recipients. New York: Berghahm Books, 2005.

LAPLANCHE, Jean; PONTALIS, Jean-Bertrand. *Vocabulary of psychoanalysis.* São Paulo: Martins Fontes, 2001.

LAQUEUR, Thomas. *Inventing sex:* body and gender from the Greeks to Freud. Rio de Janeiro: Relume Dumará, 2001, p.3-39.

LEITE, Eduardo Oliveira. *Artificial procreation and the law:* medical, religious, psychological, ethical and legal aspects. São Paulo: Ed. Revista dos Tribunais, 1995. p. 201-203.

. DNA testing, or the boundary between the genitor and the father. In: LEITE, E. O. (Coord.). *Grandes temas da actualidade:* DNA como meio de prova da filiação. Rio de Janeiro: Forense, 2000. p. 61-85.

LÉVI-STRAUSS, Claude. Introduction to the work of Mareei Mauss. In: MAUSS, Mareei. *Sociology and anthropology.* São Paulo: EDUSP, 1974. p. 1-36.

LÔWY, liana; ROUCH, Hélène. *La distinction entre sexe etgenre-,* une histoire entre biologie et culture. Paris: LHarmattan, 2003.

LUNA, Naara. Denatured motherhood: an analysis of surrogacy and egg donation. *Cadernos Pagu*, Rio de Janeiro, v. 19, p. 233-278, 2002.

. *Kinship with or without a gene: an inventory of the recent development of new reproductive technologies.* Paper presented at the XXIII Brazilian Anthropology Meeting, Research Forum 'Body, illness and sexuality', Gramado, 2002a.

. *Provetas e clones-,* uma antropologia das novas tecnologias reprodutivas. Rio de Janeiro: Fiocruz, 2007. 300p.

MACEDO, Juliana Lopes de. Defining the indefinable: considerations on the beginning of life. In: ALLEBRANDT, Débora; MACEDO, Juliana Lopes de (Org.). *Fabricating life'.* ethical, cultural and social implications of the use of new reproductive technologies. Porto Alegre: Metrópole, 2007. p. 127-143.

. et al. Profile of users of a public assisted reproduction service. In: ALLEBRANDT,

Débora; MACEDO, Juliana Lopes de (Org.). *Fabricating life* - ethical, cultural and social implications of the use of new reproductive technologies. Porto Alegre: Metrópole, 2007. p. 37-50.

MAGNANI, José Guilherme. *Brazil in the new era.* Rio de Janeiro: Zahar, 2000. 64p.

MANUEL, Czyba. La ressemblance de Fenfant né par insémination artificielle avec donneur *P* sonpère stérile. *Psychanalyse à l'Université,* n. 7, n. 28, p. 631-643, Sep. 1982.

MARCUS-STEIFF, Joachim. La Fiv's success rates: false transparencies and real messages. *La Recherche,* v. 21, n. 225, p. 1300-1312, Oct. 1990.

MARTINS, Paulo Henrique. *Contra a desumanização da medicina-,* crítica sociológica das práticas médicas modernas. Petrópolis: Vozes, 2003, 335p.

- *The gift among the moderns.* Petrópolis, Vozes, 2002.

. The sociology of Mareei Mauss: gift, symbolism and association. *Revista Crítica de Ciências Sociais,* Coimbra, n. 73, p. 45-66, Dec. 2005.

MAUSS, M. Essay on the gift: form and reason of exchange in archaic societies. In: . *Sociology and Anthropology.* São Paulo: Edusp, 1974. 239p.

MELAMED, Rose Marie M.; QUAYLE, Julieta (Org.). *Psicologia em reprodução assistida-,* experiências brasileiras. São Paulo: Casa do Psicólogo, 2006. p. 273.

MELHUUS, Marit. Exchange matters: issue of law and the flow of human substances. In: ERILSEN, T. H. *Globalisation studies in anthropology.* São Paulo: Cosac-Naify, 2003.

MELLO, Luiz. *New families-,* homosexual conjugality in contemporary Brazil. Rio de Janeiro: Garamond, 2005a.

MELO, Roberto. Gender and race in a magazine: a debate with the editors of Raça Brasil magazine. *Cadernos Pagu*, Campinas, n.6/7, 1996.

MONTEIRO, Yasmine M. Carneiro. A look at conceptions of motherhood based on new reproductive technologies in Orkut communities. In: ALLEBRANDT, Débora; MACEDO, Juliana Lopes de (Org.) *Fabricating life:* ethical, cultural and social implications of the use of new reproductive technologies. Porto Alegre: Metrópole, 2007. p. 115-126.

MOURA, Fernando Galvão; CENEDEZE, Patrícia de Felício. Semen banks in conflict with the federal constitution and the child and adolescent statute. *Paradigma,* Ribeirão Preto, v. 10, n. 11, p. 125-133, 2001.

MOURA, Simone Rolim de. Making life (for some): a debate on homosexual parenting and new reproductive technologies. In: ALLEBRANDT, Débora; MACEDO, Juliana Lopes de (Org.) *Fabricating life:* ethical, cultural and social implications of the use of new reproductive technologies. Porto Alegre: Metrópole, 2007. p. 51-66.

NASCIMENTO, Pedro. Paying the price: an ethnography of access to public assisted reproduction services in Porto Alegre/RS. In: ALLEBRANDT, Débora; MACEDO, Juliana Lopes de (Org.). *Fabricating life:* ethical, cultural and social implications of the use of new reproductive technologies. Porto Alegre: Metrópole, 2007. p. 83-104.

NUNES, Brasilmar Ferreira. The gift paradigm and medical practice. *Sociedade e Estado,* Brasília, v. 19, n. 2, jul./dez. 2004. p. 473-478.

OLIVEIRA, Cheyla Aparecida; BRAUNER, Maria Claudia Crespo. Good faith as a source of the doctor's duty of conduct in the case of assisted human reproduction. In: ALLEBRANDT, Débora; MACEDO, Juliana Lopes de (Org.) *Fabricating life:* ethical, cultural and social implications of the use of new reproductive technologies. Porto Alegre: Metrópole, 2007. p. 139154.

OLIVEIRA, Marta. On the health of the black Brazilian population. *Perspectives on Health and Reproductive Rights,* n. 4, year 2, 2001.

For over-5s, adoption is almost impossible. *Folha de São Paulo,* São Paulo, p. C-2, 26 May 2002.

PARKER, Richard. Sexual diversity, sexual analysis and AIDS education in Brazil. In: LOYOLA, Maria Andréa. *AIDS e sexualidade:* o ponto de vista das ciências humanas. Rio de Janeiro: Relume-Dumará, 1994.

PASSOS, Eduardo Pandolfi. The history of assisted reproduction: lessons learnt and future challenges. In: ALLEBRANDT, Débora; MACEDO, Juliana Lopes de (Org.). *Fabricating life:* ethical, cultural and social implications of the use of new reproductive technologies. Porto Alegre: Metrópole, 2007. p. 155-162.

PASSOS, Maria Consuêlo. The family is no longer the same: some indicators for thinking about its transformations. FERES-CARNEIRO, Terezinha (Org.). *Família e casal:* arranjos *e* demandas contemporâneas. Rio de Janeiro: Loyola, 2003. p. 13-25.

. Homoparenting: one of the other ways of being a family. *Psicologia Clínica,* Rio de Janeiro, v. 17, n. 2, p. 31-40, 2005.

RAMÍREZ-GÁLVEZ, Martha Celia. *Exclusions and displacements',* assisted reproduction and child adoption. Post-doctoral research report. São Paulo: Cebrap, 2006.

F *Children of the laboratory, luxury goods:* the commodification of reproduction. 2002. Paper presented at the XXIII Brazilian Anthropology Meeting, Gramado, June 2002.

N *New conceptive reproductive technologies:* manufacturing life, manufacturing the future. 2003. 259f. Thesis (Doctorate) - Institute of Philosophy and Human Sciences, State University of Campinas, Campinas, 2003.

RAOUL-DUVAL, Anne; BERTRAND-SERVAIS, Marie; LETUR-KÔNIRSH, Hélène; FRYDMAN, René. Que sont ces enfants devenus: les enfants des procreations médicalement assistées. *Médecine/Sciences,* n. 9, p. 747-51, 1993.

LATIN AMERICAN NETWORK FOR ASSISTED REPRODUCTION. *Latin American Registry of Assisted Reproduction.* Available at: http://www.redlara.com/registro/htm. Accessed on: 24/11/2008, at 2:28 pm.

RICHARDSON, Roberto Jarry et al. *Pesquisa social:* métodos e técnicas. São Paulo: Atlas, 1999. 334p.

ROHDEN, Fabíola. The construction of sexual difference in medicine. *Cadernos de Saúde Pública,* Rio de Janeiro, v. 19, supl. 2, p. 201-212, 2003.

ROUDINESCO, Elizabeth. *The family in disarray.* Rio de Janeiro: J. Zahar, 2003.

200p.

RUSSO, Jane Araújo. *The body against the word.* Rio de Janeiro: Ed. UFRJ, 1993. 23 lp.

SAHLINS, Marshall. Âge de *pierre, âge d'abondance:* economie des sociétés primitives. Paris: Gallimard, 1976. p. 73-98.

. *The use and abuse of biology:* an anthropological critique of sociobiology. Ann Arbor: University of Michigan, 1976a.

SALEM, Tania. The principle of anonymity in artificial insemination with donor (IAD). *Physis - Revista de Saúde Coletiva*, Rio de Janeiro, v. 5, n. 1, p. 33-68, 1995.

SALÉM, Tania; NOVAES, Simone. Recontextualising the embryo. *Revista Estudos Feministas*, Florianópolis, v. 3, n. 1, 1995.

SCAVONE, Lucila. Technologies: new choices, old conflicts. *Cadernos PAGU*, Campinas, n. 10, p. 83-112, 1998.

. *Motherhood and fatherhood in the technological age.* Paper presented at the VIII Luso-Afro-Brazilian Congress of Social Sciences, Coimbra, 2004. lOp. Available at:< http://www.ces.uc.pt/lab2004/inscricao/pdfs/painel29/LucilaScavone.pdf>. Accessed on: 13 August 2008.

SCHNEIDER, David. American kinship: a cultural account. Englewood Cliffs: Prentice-Hall, 1968.

SCHRAMM, Fermin Roland; PALÁCIOS, Marisa; REGO, Sérgio. Is the principalist bioethical model for analysing the morality of scientific research involving human beings still satisfactory? *Ciência e Saúde Coletiva*, Rio de Janeiro, v. 13, n. 2, p. 361-370, mar./abr. 2008.

SELLTIZ, Clairc; COOK, Stuart; WRIGHTSMAN, Laurence. *Research methods in social relations.* São Paulo: Herder, 1967.

SILVA, Natália Rodrigues da; LOPES, Maria de Fátima. Paternity and affective filiation in heterologous assisted reproduction techniques. In: INTERNATIONAL SEMINAR MAKING GENDER - BODY, VIOLENCE AND POWER, 8., 2008, Florianópolis, *Anais...* Florianópolis: UFSC/Centre for Philosophy and Human Sciences, 2008. p. 1-7. Available at:< http://www.fazendogenero8.ufsc.br/sts/ST21/Silva-Lopes_21.pdf>. Accessed on: 08 Dec. 2009.

STOLCKE, Verena. New reproductive technologies: same old fatherhood. *Reproductive and Genetic Engineering:* Journal of International Feminist Analysis, v. 1, n. 1, p. 5-19, 1988.

STRATHERN, Marilyn. Disparities of embodiment: gender models in the context of the new reproductive technologies. *Cambridge Anthropology, N.* 15, n. 2, p. 25-43, 1991.

. Displacing knowledge: technology and the consequences for kinship. In: GINSBURG, Faye G.; RAPP, Rayna (Ed.). *Conceiving the new world order.* Berkeley: University of California Press, 1995b. p. 323-345.

. *The gender of the gift* - problems with women and problems with society in Melanesia. Campinas: Ed. Unicamp, 2006. p. 19-77.

. The need for fathers, the need for mothers. *Revista Estudos Feministas*, Florianópolis, v. 3, n. 2, p. 303-329, 1995a.

. Regulation, substitution and possibility. In: EDWARDS, J. et al. *Technologies of procreation:* kinship in the age of assisted conception. 2. ed. London: Routledge, 1999. p. 171-216.

. *Reproducing the future-,* anthropology, kinship and the new reproductive technologies. Manchester: Manchester University Press, 1992. p. 64-89.

TAMANINI, Marlene. The dissemination of new reproductive technologies: some implications for research. In: ALLEBRANDT, Débora; MACEDO, Juliana Lopes de (Org.) *Fabricating life:* ethical, cultural and social implications of the use of new reproductive technologies. Porto Alegre: Metrópole, 2007. p. 105-114.

. New conceptive reproductive technologies: bioethics and controversies. *Revista Estudos Feministas,* Florianópolis, v. 12, n. 1, p. 73-107, jan./abr. 2004.

N New conceptive reproductive technologies in the light of bioethics and gender theories: couples and doctors in southern Brazil. 2003. 363 f. Thesis (Doctorate) - Centre for Philosophy and Human Sciences, Federal University of Santa Catarina, Florianópolis, 2003.

TARNOVSKI, Flavio Luiz. Is fatherhood all the same? The meanings of fatherhood for men who define themselves as homosexuals. In: PISCITELLI, Adriana; GREGORI, Maria Filomena; CARRARA, Sérgio (Org.). *Sexualidade e saberes:* convenções *e* fronteiras. Rio de Janeiro: Garamond, 2004. p. 385-414.

TESSER, Charles Dalcanale. Social medicalisation (I): the excessive success of modern epistemicide in health. *Interface - Comunicação, Saúde, Educação,* Botucatu, v. 10, n. 19. p. 6176, 2006.

TITMUSS, Richard. The *gift relationship-.* from human blood to social policy. New York: Vintage, 1972. p. 210-245.

TURRA, Cleusa; VENTURI, Gustavo. *Racismo cordial-,* the most complete analysis of colour prejudice in Brazil. São Paulo: Ática, 1995.

UZIEL, Anna Paula. *Family and homosexuality* - old questions, new problems. 2002. Thesis (Doctorate in Social Sciences) - Institute of Philosophy and Human Sciences, State University of Campinas, Campinas, 2002.

VIEIRA, Fernanda Bittencourt. *The technologies of reproduction* - discourses on maternity and paternity in the field of assisted reproduction in Brazil. 2008. Thesis (Doctorate in Sociology) - Institute of Social Sciences, University of Brasília, Brasília, 2008.

VÍCTORA, Ceres Gomes; KNAUTH, Daniela Ríva; HASSEN, Maria de Nazaré Agra. *Qualitative research in health.* Porto Alegre: Tomo Ed., 2000. p. 133.

YVON, Englert; SERENA, Emiliani; PHILIPPE, Revelard; FABIENNE, Devreker; CHANTAL, Laruelle; ANNE, Delbaere. *Sperm and oocyte donation:* gamete donor issues. *International Congress Series,* n. 1266, p. 303-310, Apr. 2004.

ANNEX A - Resolution no. 1.358/92 of the CFM - Federal Council of Medicine

CFM RESOLUTION N° 1.358, OF 11 November 1992.

THE **FEDERAL COUNCIL OF MEDICINE,** using the powers conferred on it by Law No. 3.268 of 30 September 1957, regulated by Decree 44.045 of 19 July 1958, and

CONSIDERING the importance of human infertility as a health problem, with medical and psychological implications, and the legitimacy of the desire to overcome it;

WHEREAS advances in scientific knowledge have already made it possible to solve many cases of human infertility;

WHEREAS Assisted Reproduction techniques have made it possible to procreate in various circumstances in which this was not possible through traditional procedures;

CONSIDERING the need to harmonise the use of these techniques with the principles of medical ethics;

CONSIDERING, finally, what was decided at the Plenary Session of the Federal Council of Medicine held on 11 November 1992;

RESOLVE

Art. I° - To adopt the ETHICAL STANDARDS FOR THE USE OF ASSISTED REPRODUCTION TECHNIQUES, annexed to this Resolution, as a deontological device to be followed by doctors.

Art. 2° - This Resolution enters into force on the date of its publication.

São Paulo-SP, 11th November 1992.

IVAN DE ARAÚJO MOURA FÉ
President

HERCULES SIDNEI PIRES LIBERAL Secretary General

Published in the Official Gazette on 19 November 1992 - Section I Page 16053.

ETHICAL STANDARDS FOR THE USE OF ASSISTED REPRODUCTION TECHNIQUES

I - GENERAL PRINCIPLES

1 - Assisted Reproduction (ART) techniques have the role of helping to solve human infertility problems, facilitating the process of procreation when other therapies have been ineffective or inefficient in resolving the current infertility situation.

2 - AR techniques can be used as long as there is an effective probability of success and there is no serious health risk for the patient or the possible offspring.

3-0 Informed consent will be mandatory and extended to infertile patients and donors. The medical aspects involving all the circumstances of the application of an ART technique will be explained in detail, as well as the results already obtained in that treatment unit with the proposed technique. The information should also include biological, legal, ethical and economic data. The informed consent document will be on a special form, and will be completed with the written agreement of the patient or infertile couple.

4 - AR techniques should not be applied with the intention of selecting the sex or any other biological characteristic of the future child, except when it comes to avoiding diseases linked to the sex of the child to be born.

5 - It is forbidden to fertilise human oocytes for any purpose other than human procreation.

6-0 The ideal number of oocytes and pre-embryos to be transferred to the recipient should be no more than four, so as not to increase the already existing risks of multiparity.

7 - In the case of multiple pregnancies resulting from the use of AR techniques, the use of procedures aimed at embryo reduction is prohibited.

II - USERS OF RA TECHNIQUES

1 - Any woman who is capable under the terms of the law, who has requested it and whose indication does not deviate from the limits of this Resolution, can be a recipient of AR techniques, provided that she has freely and knowingly agreed to it in an informed consent document.

2 - If you are married or in a stable union, you will need the approval of your spouse or partner, after a similar process of informed consent.

111 - REFERRING TO CLINICS, CENTRES OR SERVICES THAT APPLY RADIATION THERAPY TECHNIQUES.

Clinics, centres or services that apply AR techniques are responsible for controlling infectious-contagious diseases, collecting, handling, preserving, distributing and transferring human biological material to the user of AR techniques, and must meet the following minimum requirements:

1 - a person responsible for all medical and laboratory procedures carried out, who must be a doctor.

2 - a permanent record (obtained through information observed or reported by a competent source) of pregnancies, births and malformations of foetuses or newborns resulting from the different AR techniques applied in the unit in question, as well as laboratory procedures for handling gametes and pre-embryos.

3 - a permanent record of the diagnostic tests to which the human biological material that will be transferred to users of AR techniques is subjected, with the primary aim of preventing the transmission of diseases.

IV - DONATION OF GAMETES OR PRE-EMBRYOS

1 - The donation will never be for profit or commercial gain.

2 - Donors must not know the identity of recipients, and vice versa.

3 - The identity of gamete and pre-embryo donors and recipients must be kept

confidential. In special situations, information about donors may be provided exclusively to doctors for medical reasons, with the donor's civil identity being protected.

4 - Clinics, centres or services that use donation must keep a permanent record of general clinical data, phenotypic characteristics and a sample of cellular material from donors.

5 - In the region where the unit is located, the registration of pregnancies will prevent a donor from having produced more than two (2) pregnancies, of different sexes, in an area of one million inhabitants.

6 - The choice of donors is the responsibility of the unit. As far as possible, it should ensure that the donor has the greatest phenotypic and immunological similarity and the greatest possibility of compatibility with the recipient.

7 - The doctor in charge of the clinics, units or services, or the members of the multidisciplinary team who provide services there, will not be allowed to participate as donors in the AR programmes.

V - CRYOPRESERVATION OF GAMETES OR PRE-EMBRYOS

1 - Clinics, centres or services may cryopreserve sperm, eggs and pre-embryos.

2-0 the total number of pre-embryos produced in the laboratory will be communicated to the patients, so that they can decide how many pre-embryos will be transferred fresh, and the surplus will be

cryopreserved and cannot be discarded or destroyed.

3 - At the time of cryopreservation, the spouses or partners must express their wishes in writing as to the fate of the cryopreserved pre-embryos in the event of divorce, serious illness or the death of one or both of them, and when they wish to donate them.

VI - DIAGNOSIS AND TREATMENT OF PRE-EMBRYOS

AR techniques can also be used to preserve and treat genetic or hereditary diseases, when perfectly indicated and with sufficient diagnostic and therapeutic guarantees.

1 - Any intervention on pre-embryos "in vitro" for diagnostic purposes cannot have any other purpose than the assessment of their viability or the detection of hereditary diseases, and the informed consent of the couple is mandatory.

2 - Any intervention for therapeutic purposes on "in vitro" pre-embryos will have no other purpose than to treat a disease or prevent its transmission, with real guarantees of success, and the informed consent of the couple is mandatory.

3-0 The maximum development time for "in vitro" pre-embryos is 14 days.

VII - ON SURROGATE PREGNANCY (TEMPORARY DONATION OF THE UTERUS)

Clinics, centres or human reproduction services can use AR techniques to create the situation identified as surrogate pregnancy, as long as there is a medical problem that prevents or contraindicates pregnancy in the genetic donor.

1 - Temporary uterus donors must belong to the family of the genetic donor, up to the second degree of kinship, and other cases are subject to authorisation by the Regional Medical Council.

2 - The temporary donation of the uterus cannot be of a lucrative or commercial nature.

ANNEX B - Informed consent form

I, , R.G: , hereby declare that I have agreed to be interviewed for the field research entitled "Assisted reproduction: a study on semen donation in the Brazilian context", carried out by the Institute of Social Medicine (IMS) of the State University of Rio de Janeiro (UERJ). I have also been informed that the research is being coordinated by Ana Paula Cavalcante dos Santos, whom I can contact/consult at any time I deem necessary via telephone numbers (21) 3511-2472 and 9265-5900 or via e-mail: *pesquisa_doacao@ims.uerj.br and .pesquisadoacaodesemen@gmail.com*

I state that I agreed to take part of my own free will, without receiving any financial incentive and for the sole purpose of collaborating in the success of the research. I have been informed of the strictly academic aims of the study, which, in general terms, are to characterise the motivating factors for semen donation.

I was also informed that the use of the information I have provided is subject to the ethical standards for research involving human beings of the National Research Ethics Commission (CONEP) of the National Health Council of the Ministry of Health.

My collaboration will be anonymous, by means of a semi-structured interview in the first stage and a focus group in the second stage, the meetings of which will be recorded as soon as this authorisation is signed. The data collected will only be accessed and analysed by the researcher, her supervisor (Prof. Luiz Antonio de Castro Santos) and her co-supervisor (Maria Helena Rodrigues Navas Zarnora).

I am aware that, should I have any doubts or feel harmed, I can contact the researcher responsible, or her supervisors, or the Research Ethics Committee of the Institute of Social Medicine of UERJ (CEP-IMS), located at Rua São Francisco Xavier, 524 - sala 7.003-D, Maracanã, Rio de Janeiro (RJ), CEP 20559-900, telephone (x-21) 2587-7303 ext. 248 or 232 and fax (x-21) 2264-1142.

The principal investigator of the study provided me with a signed copy of this Free and Informed Consent Form on today's date, in accordance with the recommendations of the National Research Ethics Commission (CONEP).

I have also been informed that I can withdraw from this research with just one communication to the researcher in charge, at any time, without any damage, sanctions or embarrassment.

Rio de Janeiro, 2009

Participant's signature

____

Researcher's signature

____

Ana Paula Cavalcante dos Santos

PhD student at IMS/UERJ - Registration DO XXXiii

ANNEX C - Interview script

Research: Semen donation in the Brazilian context.
Main research question: *motivation for semen donation.*

PART I - Personal data:

Name:
Age:
Age of Donation:
Nationality:
Marital status:
Do you have children?
Profession:
Occupation:
Religion:
Income:
Family income:
Where you live:
Date of interview:

Duration:

PART II - Topics guiding the research.

a. Your level of knowledge about CRTs and gamete donation.

b. Opinion on practice.

c. Main motivating factor for semen donation.

d. Experience with the donation process/contact with the semen bank.

e. Donor profile. Do you regularly donate in other ways?

f. Social relations and semen donation.

g. Knowledge of TRC regulations and gamete donation.

h. Opinion on the rules of anonymity and gratuity.

i. How do you think/feel about the fate of your semen after collecting the material: bank/lab - freezing - recipient - pregnancy - birth.

j. Representation of his son.

k. How do you deal with the child born from donated gametes?

l. Position on the use of one's own semen by heterosexual and homosexual couples, single women and older people.

m. Would you use donated semen in case of infertility?

n. Religious formation.

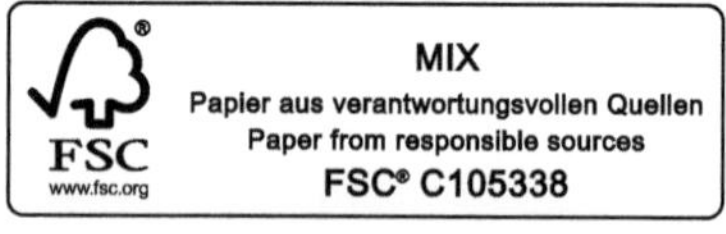

Printed by Books on Demand GmbH, Norderstedt / Germany